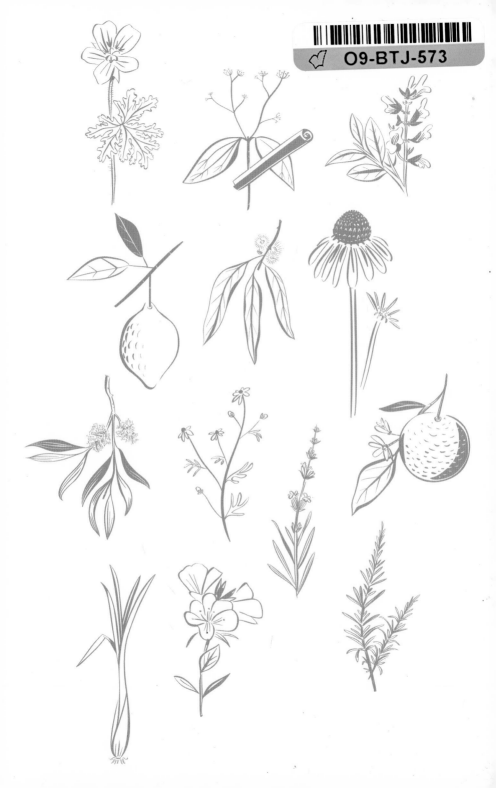

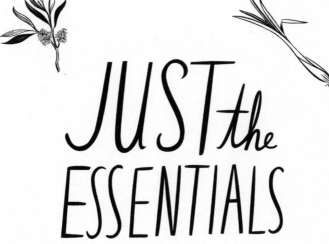

JUST the ESSENTIALS

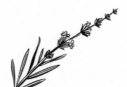

Also by Adina Grigore

SKIN CLEANSE

JUST the ESSENTIALS

HOW ESSENTIAL OILS CAN HEAL YOUR SKIN, IMPROVE YOUR HEALTH, and DETOX YOUR LIFE

Adina Grigore

HARPER WAVE

An Imprint of HarperCollinsPublishers

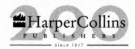

This book contains advice and information relating to health care. It should be used to supplement rather than replace the advice of your doctor or another trained health professional. If you know or suspect you have a health problem, it is recommended that you seek your physician's advice before embarking on any medical program or treatment. All efforts have been made to ensure the accuracy of the information contained in this book as of the date of publication. This publisher and the author disclaim liability for any medical outcomes that may occur as a result of applying the methods suggested in this book.

FIRST EDITION

Illustrations by Libby VanderPloeg
Designed by William Ruoto

Library of Congress Cataloging-in-Publication Data has been applied for.

ISBN 978-0-06-244891-0

17 18 19 20 21   RRD   10 9 8 7 6 5 4 3 2

Dedicated to everyone who patiently helped with my essential oil detective work.

Contents

Introduction   xi

Part I: The 101   **1**

Chapter 1   Essential Oils Are Awesome   3

Chapter 2   A History Lesson   13

Chapter 3   The Big Business of Essential Oils   23

Part II: How to Harness the Amazing Benefits of Essential Oils   **35**

Chapter 4   Essential Oils Stripped Down   37

Chapter 5   But What Do I Do with Them?   51

Chapter 6   Making Sense of Essential Oil Jargon   75

Chapter 7   The Beginner's Top Ten   87

Chapter 8   It's Time to DIY   117

Conclusion   187

Essential Oil FAQs   189

Acknowledgments   193

Notes   195

Index   209

Introduction

Hello, and welcome to the only book about essential oils you'll ever need. How do I know that? Because at this point in my natural-beauty journey, I've pretty much read them all.

Let me explain.

I'm a super-normal girl, not some massive hippie (just an ordinary one), not a dermatologist, and not an aromatherapist. What I am is someone with extremely sensitive skin. If you've read my book *Skin Cleanse*, then you already know this story (feel free to turn to Chapter 1 now), but for most of my life, I struggled with chronic skin issues—constant rashes, acne, painful redness—and could never find lasting relief. Even after I did a pretty good job of cleaning up my diet and lifestyle, my skin remained a mess. I tried every new product available, thinking that maybe I just wasn't washing, toning, or moisturizing in a way that was "right for my skin type." And when that didn't work I went to all the doctors and dermatologists I could and slathered myself in steroid creams and prescription shampoos and gobbled up antibiotics and acne pills. You know what happened? Nothing. Just more itchy, inflamed skin.

It was like I was lost in a black hole, and I felt so bad about myself. No matter what I tried, my skin wasn't getting any better. So one day I just . . . gave up. Just like that. I stopped everything—my medications, my makeup and skincare products, my shampoo and conditioner, and my doctors' appointments. I was exhausted. I just wanted a break from it all. So I spent a few days washing with only water and using absolutely no products (I swear, it wasn't as gross as it sounds). And guess what? That's when my skin started to get better.

It took this crazy experiment born of desperation for me to realize I wasn't treating my skin with the same respect that I held for the rest of my body. And even though, as a nutritionist, I'd learned to keep a watchful eye out for synthetic chemicals and preservatives on food labels, I definitely wasn't applying the same degree of scrutiny to my beauty products.

So, I got to work educating myself on how to make my own products using whole, natural ingredients. What started out as a last-ditch attempt to heal my skin in my tiny Brooklyn kitchen has now become my full-time livelihood as the founder and CEO of the all-natural skincare line S.W. Basics. Today we're sold by some of the largest retailers in the country *and* I've met Martha Stewart in person. NBD.

And it all started with my impromptu skin cleanse.

In my journey toward better skin, I learned that the quality of your skin is only as good as the quality of your skincare—

and the quality of your skincare is only as good as the quality of its ingredients. When I switched from using formulas made from ingredients I couldn't pronounce to versions made from, say, coconut oil and sea salt, it was as if I had stumbled upon a sorcerer's chest of magical, healing elixirs. Who knew that simple, natural ingredients could do more than smell pretty and taste nice—that they contained potent plant-based compounds that offered real benefits for your skin? It seemed almost too good to be true.

Once I was hooked on the healing powers of plants, everyone started telling me I had to try essential oils. I have to admit, I was skeptical at first. This is not because I hadn't read a trillion things about how amazing they were. I had. It's because I just didn't believe it.

There's a ton of marketing hype around essential oils. A quick Internet search might leave you convinced that they'll cure everything from a blister to a terrible love life. I mean it. Type any ailment into your web browser combined with the words "essential oil" and you will discover that all you've ever needed to do to be happy and healthy was diffuse some oil in your bedroom. How could you not have known that? How could we *all* not have known that?

The truth is, a lot of the claims out there about essential oils are dubious at best. Most of the information you'll find about them online is completely unverified—and possibly downright dangerous. For this reason and many others, essential oils have long suffered from an image problem. People blog about them, sell them, or your one weird aunt raves about their benefits, but most of us haven't really found reliable sources of information about how to incorporate essential oils into our lives.

As I said, I used to feel the same way about them as you

probably do now. They're super mysterious and kind of intimidating. And there are so many of them. *Where are you even supposed to start?*

As you probably guessed when you picked up this book, I now find them way less mysterious and confusing. When I was climbing my way up from rock bottom, I put aside my skepticism and decided to give essential oils a try. I'd heard that some of them were great for acne, and I'd been dealing with breakouts my whole life. In my new "less is more, especially when it comes to chemicals" philosophy, adding a few drops of essential oils to my homemade products seemed like a perfect solution (that is, if they actually worked). Plus, they smelled nice—and certain natural ingredients (sorry, apple cider vinegar) can smell so decidedly not nice you're almost tempted to return to your fake oceanside-breeze-with-a-piña-colada-

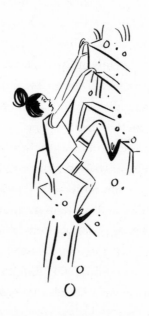

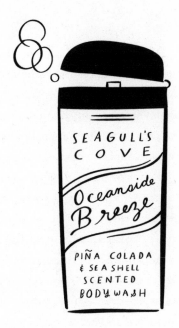

scented face wash. So I started adding essential oils to my DIY products to make them work—and smell—better.

It turns out, that's a really good way to get hooked on essential oils, and that's exactly what happened to me. I was honestly amazed by their power and efficacy. Those tiny bottles of potion improved my life (and my skin) tremendously. Today, I incorporate essential oils into my skincare and life in a ton of different ways. I've used minty oils to make toothpaste, tea tree oil to kill horrible tooth infections, eucalyptus and citronella oils to repel moths and bugs, clove oil to speed up the course of a flu, cinnamon oil to quiet a migraine, and lemon oil to clean my counters. My beauty cabinet houses more essential oils than any other product. In fact, essential oils are my first line of

THE DIY DETOX

One reason you may have picked up this book is that you're concerned about the amount of chemicals present in your life. And the fact is, most of our homes and workspaces and bodies are now contaminated by any number of toxic substances. Think about some of the chemicals you encounter every day. Household bleach is an insanely dangerous chemical and the number-one cause of poisoning in the United States—it's contained in many common laundry detergents and bathroom cleaners. We use degreasers for our dishes that contain petroleum distillates (aka by-products of gasoline), which are known to irritate lung tissue and nerve cells, and glass cleaners with ammonia, which irritates the skin, eyes, and respiratory system. Much of our food is genetically modified and/or treated with pesticides, and then we store our leftovers in plastic derived from more petroleum byproducts that can leach into our foods and can cause hormone dysfunction.

The vast majority of our skincare products contain preservatives, fillers, and synthetic fragrances. All of these chemicals—considered "safe" by government standards—have been linked to multiple types of cancer, genital deformities, obesity, diabetes, and infertility. Even tampons release formaldehyde (which is a toxin linked to cancer) directly into your bloodstream.

I don't like to dwell too much on these frightening facts because a scared DIYer is not a happy DIYer, and I really do want to encourage you to have fun with essential oils. But I think that knowing or even just being reminded of the amount of chemicals present in our daily lives is a great way to feel empowered to make simple changes that can significantly lessen your toxic load. Making your own products from natural ingredients is one easy way to help protect yourself and your family from everyday exposures to scary chemicals.

defense for many things. When it comes to S.W. Basics, essential oils are the rock star ingredients that make our products even more potent, delicious-smelling, and shelf-stable.

So stick around. If you've heard the hype and it sounds too good to be true; if you use one or two oils but don't know how to get into other ones; if you use natural skincare with essential oils but have no idea why or what they're doing for you, this is where you're finally going to get some answers. First, we're going to have a lesson in essential oils: What are they exactly, and why should you care? After the 101, we'll look at the properties and benefits of specific oils, and how you can go about finding the ones that will work for you. Then we're going to get crafty together, so that you end up with everything you need to easily incorporate essential oils into your everyday life.

At the very least, I want you to understand the incredibly wide-ranging and potent benefits of these all-natural, plant-based ingredients. That's what this book is here for. I'm not going to make you feel like you need to become an herbalist, or overhaul your entire beauty cabinet, or get so into essential oils that you lose your friends (although if that happens, call me and I'll hire you to come work at S.W. Basics). Instead, I want to share what I've learned about them, guide you toward finding your favorites, and show you how to use them. Maybe you'll start making your own perfume. Maybe you'll come up with a killer laundry detergent and start your own company (or gift it to all of your friends who are using terrible alternatives). Maybe you'll help patchouli make a comeback in your town. I'm into any or all of these outcomes.

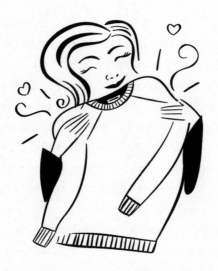

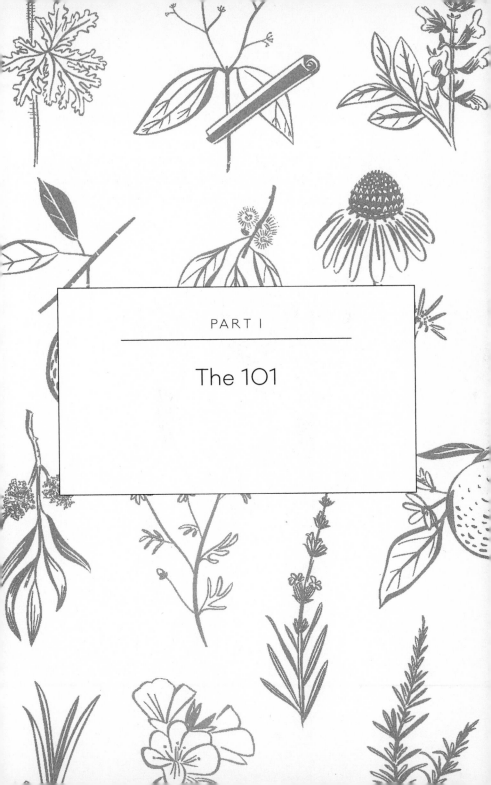

PART I

The 101

CHAPTER 1

Essential Oils Are Awesome

B ut deep down you already knew that. You picked up this book because you had a hunch that essential oils might change your life. And you were correct.

For some of you, it's possible that this isn't your first foray into the world of essential oils. Perhaps you were derailed when the information available online seemed too outlandish, or when the other books out there required you to have a chemistry degree or a soul from the 1970s to get through them.

I get it. But let me tell you, you've been missing out. Not in the sense that you haven't been enjoying the positive effects of essential oils in your life—they are all around you whether you know it or not. But isn't it kind of sad that these amazing little plant-based powerhouses have been all but invisible to you?

(And that, perhaps, you're even a little bit scared of them?) I'm here to stop that doubt and fear in its tracks. Consider me the new PR person for essential oils, because I want to give them a makeover and turn them into stars. If essential oils were a baby Justin Bieber, I would be their Usher.

Why Essential Oils Are Right for You

To start, there is actually plenty of scientific evidence that not only are essential oils *not* scary, but they are in fact quite beneficial for your health.

There are two main reasons why you don't often hear about this research. The first is that there's still much to be investigated (Mother Nature is pretty epic and complex). The second reason is that the results of most reliable studies are funneled into research used to create patented drugs rather than to commercialize love for plants. For example, when was the last time you saw an ad for willow bark on the back of a city bus? Now, how about the last time you saw an ad for aspirin—which is derived from the *Salix* (willow) tree? Didn't realize the connection? Thought so. Major pharmaceutical companies often bankroll essential oils research, but since natural plant substances cannot easily be patented, there is less potential profit in them—and consequently less funding for their development and promotion. But that doesn't mean the research doesn't exist. It's just been waiting for me to come along and tell you all about it.

So you might not be seeing them in Super Bowl ads just yet (can't wait!), but that doesn't mean essential oils aren't *everywhere*. I guarantee that many of them are already a part of your daily routine. In fact, you might be shocked to learn just how important a role many essential oils have played not only in your life, but in the evolution of our society.

For one thing, essential oils are quite literally the foundational elements of contemporary medicine. Beginning thousands of years ago and across a range of cultures—the ancient civilizations of Egypt, China, India, and Rome, to name a few—essential oils were critical elements in healing and wellness rites. Hippocrates, "the Father of Medicine," meticulously examined the effects of oils from more than three hundred plants, famously saying, "A perfumed bath and a scented massage every day is the way to good health."

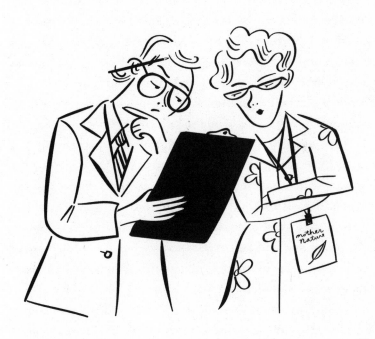

Even as science and technology have advanced, researchers continually turn to Mother Nature (the first and ultimate chemist) for inspiration when developing synthetic drugs. Many of today's most common medicines—from codeine to morphine, Vicks VapoRub to lice spray—are derived from plant oils and extracts. So even if you're the biggest skeptic out there when it comes to "natural medicine," if you've taken any prescription or over-the-counter drug in your lifetime, chances are you've reaped the benefits of essential oils.

Those benefits extend into the rest of your life, too. For instance, essential oils are the predecessors of all synthetic fragrance. Every lavender-scented dish soap, rose-smelling moisturizer, or cinnamon-laced lip balm you've ever used is a *direct imitation* of the OG, essential oil. Essential oils are also the basis for natural flavorings, which can be found in products ranging from toothpaste to orange juice. Essential oils are all around you, and they have been for a very, very long time.

But essential oils are not just sweet-smelling (or -tasting) liquids. They're some of the most potent, concentrated, and effective parts of a plant, distilled into a hyperconcentrated form. Pure essential oils are composed of the super-fuel of a plant, which has tremendous implications for you and me. Depending on the oil, their properties can include antimicrobial, antibacterial, analgesic (aka painkilling), antiseptic, antispasmodic, and anti-inflammatory benefits (don't worry, we'll go into detail on all of this soon!). They can help boost the immune system and promote circulation. They can provide soothing, mood-enhancing effects and, in some cases, may help to alleviate depression. And while research is ongoing, they could even turn out to be effective tools in the fight against cancer.

We will discuss in detail all of these amazing properties and more. By the end of this book, I promise you that you'll be in awe of the magic of plant extracts. And you don't need to be sick to benefit from them. You can use them day in and day out as preventive care to enhance your health. They are incredibly egalitarian: they can enhance the lives of *everyone*, from the free spirit at Burning Man who wants to, you know, *just relax, man* to the high-powered executive looking for a natural way to treat her tension headaches to the busy mom seeking a safer alternative to chemical-laden home products. And while they might seem like a niche commodity, when you start to look more closely, you'll see that they're both easy to find and superaffordable. With just a little bit of information (in the form of this kickass book) you can begin reaping their rewards immediately.

And there are so many rewards. Essential oils can be used to treat aches and pains; they can be employed as potent, natural cleaning detergents. They are proven repellents for mosquitoes and can help alleviate the symptoms of skin ailments like dandruff and eczema. On a purely superficial level, many smell amazing and make wonderful fragrances. On a deeper level, they can be integrated into alternative healing modalities in order to improve the quality of your health (completely naturally, I might add). I mean, what other tools do you have so readily at your disposal that offer all of these benefits *and* all of this creativity? Yep, that's what I thought.

Seriously: whether you're interested in health, wellness, science, nature, history, anthropology, medicine, physiology, or art, I'm pretty sure that you will find essential oils both helpful and fun. So, basically, no matter who you are, you're also going to find this book really helpful and fun. I promise. Let's get this party started, shall we?

The EO Origin Story

All most of us know about essential oils is that they're those strange, smelly liquids in little dark bottles sold at the health food store. And if you don't shop at health food stores, even that might be more than you know about them.

So what the eff are essential oils anyway? And where do they come from?

Thanks to their name, a lot of people think of essential oils as the "essence" of a plant, and that's a nice way to consider them. Plant "essence" sounds kind of magical, like something a wizard would use to create healing potions. Which, honestly, isn't that far off the mark, because essential oils are derived from a little-understood and kind of magical part of plants.

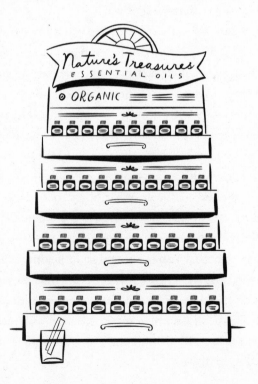

All plants produce two types of compounds that are crucial to the plant's survival. One is primary metabolites, which help support the plant's growth and development. Metabolites include cellulose, which gives plants structure, and starch, which gives them energy and helps them grow. Primary metabolites keep plants alive.

HYDROSOL

Throughout this text, you'll occasionally see the term "hydrosol." Put simply, a hydrosol is sort of like a water-diluted version of a pure essential oil. In steam distillation (one common way in which plant oils are extracted), a mixture of steam and essential oil and water-soluble plant compounds flows into a tube where condensation occurs. The liquid is captured in a separate vessel where two byproducts emerge: essential oil and the plant water, or hydrosol. This liquid is infused with plant material, and can contain powerful compounds.

Let's use lavender as an example. Its hydrosol not only possesses the plant's signature aroma, but it also contains the soothing, anti-inflammatory properties associated with lavender, in a less concentrated form than in its essential oil. I consider hydrosols to be wonderful complements to essential oils. I incorporate hydrosols into my routine often and find that they make great bases for skincare because they're incredibly gentle. I'm going to teach you how to make your own hydrosol, and in Chapter 8, I'll provide some simple recipes that integrate hydrosols. I encourage you to give them a try!

The other necessary compounds are called secondary metabolites. These help the plant survive in its environment. For instance, secondary metabolites attract pollinators or repel the bugs who want to eat the plant. Lots of times these secondary metabolites are what give a plant its striking color and strong smell or flavor. Alkaloids are a kind of secondary metabolite that make a plant taste bad and sometimes actually poison and kill whoever (or whatever) might want to consume it. Morphine and codeine (derived from opium poppy seeds) and cocaine are alkaloids. So are caffeine and nicotine. (Leave it to humans to turn a plant's chemical warfare resources into recreational drugs.) Whether they relax or stimulate the nervous system, all of these plant-produced metabolites work to ward off the insects and animals that would eat the plant or, on the flip side, to attract the ones that would pollinate it, helping it reproduce. Even though scientists know a lot about secondary metabolites, they've just barely scratched the surface in understanding the full scope of what they can do for the plants that produce them.

One of the more mysterious secondary metabolites is—uh, you guessed it—a plant's essential oil. More than likely, essential oils operate in a way very similar to other secondary metabolites: they protect the plant by harming predators or attracting pollinators. The most obvious way they do this is through smell. Essential oils create the powerful smells we associate with plants, and these smells function to attract or deter animals. Attracting the right animals, like bees, helps the plant cross-pollinate. Alternatively, the strong smell can keep predators away. Some essential oils can actually produce neurotoxic effects, particularly in insects, so these oils are like very tiny, very badass bodyguards. It is also possible that, in some plants, essential oils help heal and protect the plant physically, by sealing wounds, acting as a varnish to keep water in rather than letting it evaporate (so the plant stays hydrated and nourished), and providing backup energy for the plant when it isn't receiving enough carbon dioxide. Some essential oils act as a plant's perspiration, or transpiration—they travel through the leaves and out of the "pores" of the leaves, then evaporate into the atmosphere.

Personally, I think this information is fascinating—essential oils have so many functions in nature, all to keep a plant alive! Think about all of the ways they might be able to benefit us.

QUICK FACTS ABOUT ESSENTIAL OILS

- All plants produce essential oils in varying quantities. The oils you see on the market are derived from plants that produce enough oil to cultivate. This helps explain why you can easily find some essential oils (like lavender) for just a few bucks a bottle while others (like sandalwood) are much harder to find and superexpensive. Lavender is a much more widely cultivated crop than sandalwood and it takes a lot less plant material to process the same quantity of oil.
- Some plants simply don't make enough oil to be bottled on their own at all. Witch hazel, for example, produces very little oil—so it's sold only as a hydrosol (see box on page 130 for more information on hydrosols).

- An essential oil is different from other plant oils (like olive or coconut oil) in that it doesn't offer nutritive value. Instead, it is made up of what are called "volatile components," which simply means they easily evaporate into the air. These compounds are what give the plant its scent and flavor.
- Technically, an essential oil is a plant extract, though when you see "extract" on a label, it is much less potent and less concentrated than an essential oil, and usually used for flavoring.
- An essential oil is seventy to eighty times stronger than its herbal counterpart. For example, you would need to drink more than twenty-eight cups of peppermint tea to match the potency of one drop of peppermint oil.

It's a little frustrating that there's still so much we don't understand about exactly how essential oils function to protect the plants that produce them—because the more we understand about their protective role in plant life, the more we can understand their potential to benefit human life. But the fact that we know about only a fraction of their benefits is also kind of cool if you think about it. Plant oils have so much power that we can barely fathom their impact on us. Like water and air, they are the basis of life and have been recognized as such by humans for literally thousands of years. So, next, we're going to take a little journey through history to learn about all the cultures that made use of the therapeutic properties of essential oils long before we started putting them in dark little bottles.

CHAPTER 2

A History Lesson

For millennia, across the globe, people have been using essential oils for all kinds of purposes: medicinal, religious, cosmetic, and culinary, to name just a few. Given the wide variety of uses for essential oils—and the fact that we've been using them for such a long time—it's surprising how underutilized and misunderstood they remain today. Let's take a moment to learn about the supercool history of essential oils so that we can appreciate just how interwoven they were (and are) in humanity's cultural fabric.

To begin our journey, we're heading back to the ancient societies of Egypt, Rome, Greece, Persia, India, and China. The first use of essential oils is often traced to ancient Egypt— unsurprising, given what geniuses those Egyptians were (and are). You probably know that Egyptian mathematics, astronomy, and agriculture were more sophisticated than the sciences of most other cultures at the time, but you may not know that Egyptians were just as inventive when it came to using plants to their advantage (case in point: they created the first recorded recipe for deodorant in 1500 BCE).

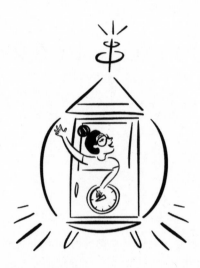

Egyptian doctors were well regarded for their extensive knowledge of plant substances, including oils. They used frankincense, sandalwood, and myrrh as insect repellents, as salves for wounds, and for dental hygiene. And Egyptian priests used plants to help treat nervousness and depression. Blue lily (often called blue lotus) was so popular among Egyptians that it is depicted in numerous hieroglyphics and has been found in high quantities in mummified bodies. (Blue lily is a hypnotic, an aphrodisiac, and a painkiller.) You could argue that the Egyptians originated aromatherapy *and* psychopharmacology.

Aside from using them as a key ingredient in medicinal treatments, the Egyptians used plant oils both in the embalming (aka mummy-making) process and extensively in religious ceremonies. They believed aromatic oils helped create a connection between human beings and the divine: Gods were often associated with sweet scents (there was even a god of perfume, Nefertem) and only royalty and high priests had ready access to the highest-quality oils. In fact, aroma played such a large role in most religious ceremonies that nearly every large sanctuary contained a dedicated perfume-producing unit.

These were, of course, not the pure essential oils that we know today. Modern methods of production hadn't yet been invented, so ancient cultures were more likely to either burn plant resins and aromatic woods to release their oils into the air or to steep herbs, flowers, resins, and fragrant woods in another oil like olive or almond or sesame, heating it until it was fully infused with the plant essence. Or they would boil the plant matter in a mixture of oil and water, then skim off the infused oil for later use.

Other ancient cultures utilized plant oils in a similar manner, taking advantage of their naturally therapeutic properties and heavenly fragrances in both medicine and religion. In Ancient India, aromatic oils and botanicals were integral elements of Ayurvedic medicine. (I'm sure you already know this from your friend who puts turmeric in everything she cooks, but Ayurveda—known as the "science of life"—is a holistic approach to health and wellness that began in India thousands of years ago and is still going strong today.) Ayurveda practitioners incorporated essences of such aromatic plants as fennel, lemongrass, patchouli, jasmine, sandalwood, clove, and (of course) turmeric to help promote healing and well-being through both topical application and aromatherapy.

OILS FOR EVERY OCCASION, ACCORDING TO YOUR ACUPUNCTURIST

My friend Giselle Wasfie is a music journalist–turned–licensed acupuncturist. She's interviewed Björk and Mos Def, but she also has a master's degree in Traditional Chinese Medicine. I asked her to share her favorite essential oils for different occasions, as well as the best places on your body to apply them according to Traditional Chinese Medicine.

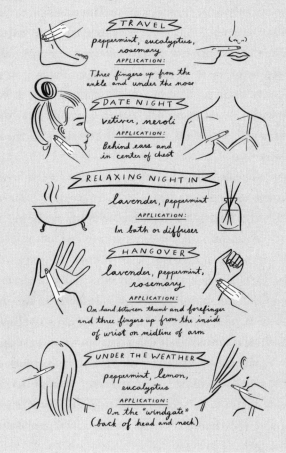

TRAVEL
peppermint, eucalyptus, rosemary
APPLICATION:
Three fingers up from the ankle and under the nose

DATE NIGHT
vetiver, neroli
APPLICATION:
Behind ears and in center of chest

RELAXING NIGHT IN
lavender, peppermint
APPLICATION:
In bath or diffuser

HANGOVER
lavender, peppermint, rosemary
APPLICATION:
On hand between thumb and forefinger and three fingers up from the inside of wrist on midline of arm

UNDER THE WEATHER
peppermint, lemon, eucalyptus
APPLICATION:
On the "windgate" (back of head and neck)

And Ancient China had it all figured out too. Many of the herbal-based treatments the Chinese developed are still thriving today. It's crazy to think that some of the plant oils that remain a big part of Traditional Chinese Medicine were already in use in roughly 2600 BCE! What's even more astonishing is the fact that the Ancient Chinese medicine cabinet included some two thousand herbs and botanical substances.

In Ancient Greece, as in Egypt, aromatic oils were linked to the spiritual realm: gods and goddesses were believed to don scented robes and the afterlife was supposedly rose-scented (which sounds pretty nice, right?). The Greek physician Hippocrates, as noted earlier, spent much of his time studying plants and oils.

Fragrant oils also make numerous appearances in both the New and the Old Testaments of the Bible. The Three Wise Men presented the newborn baby Jesus with a gift of not just gold, but also frankincense and myrrh. In one story, Jesus forgives a woman her sins after she gives him a foot massage with essential oil. (Who wouldn't have?) "Anointing oil" was created with myrrh, cinnamon, and calamus oils and is still used today in some Christian sacred rituals. Anointing oil was considered holy and was thought to prevent death—implying that people who used essential oils seemed healthier and safer. Plants and their oils were standard gifts for kings and deities. Imagine, fragrant medicinal plants good enough for Jesus and as valuable as gold! If that doesn't say something about how important plant essences were at the time, I don't know what else could.

In Ancient Rome, Pliny the Elder cited the many beneficial properties of plants in his seminal text *Natural History*, noting, for example, the various and wide-ranging uses of rosemary for well-being. Another Roman (by way of Greece), Galen of Pergamum, furthered the applications of essential oils in medicinal use by serving as personal physician to the Roman emperor Marcus Aurelius. His writings—more than 350 in total— would ultimately inspire another huge figure in the history of essential oils, Ali ibn Sina, aka Avicenna.

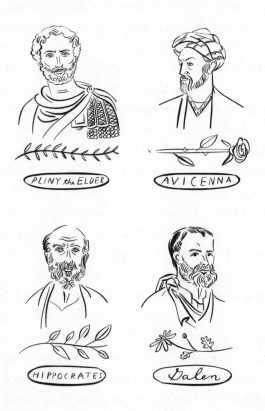

A Persian, Avicenna was heavily influenced by the medicinal theories coming out of Rome and Egypt, adding to the growing body of plant-based research with his *Canon of Medicine*—an epic treatise compiling the therapeutic uses of hundreds of plants. Even more awesome (for the purposes of this book), he was a true pioneer in the process of steam distillation for producing essential oils. While the Egyptians, Romans, and Greeks were all either burning or infusing oils to make use of plant essences, and distillation definitely existed before Avicenna came along, he really helped make it a trend. (Avicenna would have been huge on Twitter.) Today, steam distillation is one of the most widespread methods of producing essential oils.

Oh, and as if that wasn't enough, here's one more reason Avicenna gets an Essential Oil Lifetime Achievement Award: he's thought to be the first person to extract the essence of rose, which kicked off a frenzy of rose essential oil and rosewater exports from Arabia. He basically laid the groundwork for perfume as we know it today.

Meanwhile, on the other side of the world . . . long before Europeans made it over to North America, Native Americans were using echinacea for headaches, horsemint for body aches, and white pine for colds. They were well versed in the benefits of plant oils and had quite the botanical pharmacy.

The list goes on and on. As you can see, plant and essential oils were not relegated to the crusty medicine cabinets of a select few shamans, warlocks, or witches. They were used extensively in a multitude of settings by prominent physicians and pharmacists, scientists and clergymen, royals and laypeople. Moreover, their role in some of the most celebrated rituals and traditions in civilizations in history is uncontested.

As the popularity of and demand for plant oils across the world continued to grow, techniques to produce oils became increasingly sophisticated. By 1200, the Grasse region of France had established itself as the global hub of perfume making. But there were other, more urgent, uses for essential oils than perfume: with the advent of the bubonic plague, European physicians were desperate to find new ways to help heal the sick. They formulated concoctions from the oils of camphor, meadowsweet, rosemary, and lavender. Frankincense (one of the most crucial essential oils throughout history) was burned in the streets in order to eliminate illness and evil spirits. Indeed, frankincense kills germs, soothes and clears the respiratory tract, and reduces anxiety. So while we'll never know if it cured the bubonic plague (or if Harry Potter could have used it against Dementors), we do know those doctors were definitely onto something.

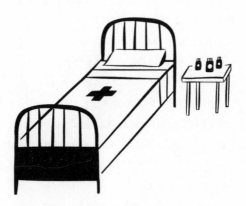

Essential oils continued to be utilized and cultivated over the centuries, with the 1653 book *Complete Herbal* by Englishman Nicholas Culpeper providing detailed recipes to address a wide range of ailments. Then, in the first half of the twentieth century, a simple accident led to a major breakthrough in our understanding and application of essential oils.

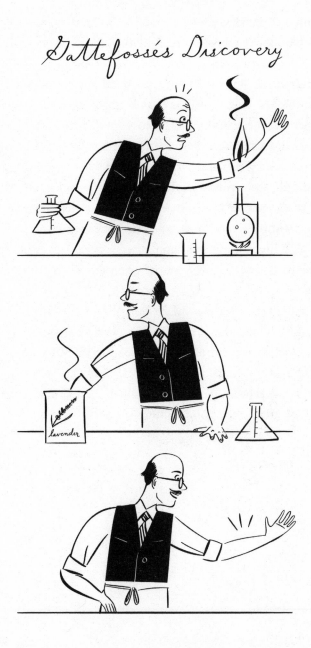

Gattefossé's Discovery

René-Maurice Gattefossé, a French chemist, was working in his laboratory when he accidentally burned his hand. Immediately, he treated the burn with lavender essential oil. He was astonished and delighted when his hand healed quickly, without any of the complications typical of the day, like infection.

That discovery inspired Gattefossé to dedicate his life's work to studying what he called "aromatherapy." He began testing essential oils on hospital patients, and in 1937 used his findings to publish the groundbreaking book *Aromathérapie*. Shortly thereafter, another Frenchman, Jean Valnet, used essential oils to successfully treat the wounds of injured soldiers in World War II. This research and application were invaluable in reinforcing the healing powers of essential oils to the medical community at large.

Right about now you might be asking yourself: If essential oils are so great, why aren't they as prevalent in our culture today as they were thousands of years ago? Why doesn't *my* doctor treat me with lavender oil? (If only Gattefossé was still around . . .) I mean, if essential oils were good enough for royalty, why aren't they good enough for us?

These are all such great questions.

CHAPTER 3

The Big Business of Essential Oils

While history clearly offers evidence of how important essential oils have been in the past, today most of us probably still think of them as fringe products. The truth is, essential oils are actually a pretty big business. They may still be flying under the mainstream radar, but they're quickly gaining traction as part of a growing industry—or actually, a huge, booming industry.

Young Living, one of the companies at the top of the essential oil food chain, reported sales of over $1 billion in 2015. (That's *buh*-billion.) And they use what's called a direct-sales model, which means you can buy Young Living essential oils only from a friend or online. In other words, a company whose products don't even appear on any shelf of any physical store is selling a billion dollars' worth of essential oil products a year. And it's not like they're the only game in town. Plenty of other essential oil purveyors (like Aura Cacia, Now, Bach, and *yes*, S.W. Basics) sell their products in stores. In fact, the entire essential oil market is growing every year and is expected to hit $11.7 billion by 2022 (and let me tell you, as an insider, I think the rate of growth is even faster than that).

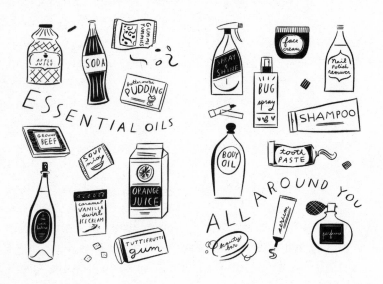

Want to know the largest wholesale accounts for essential oil manufacturers? No, it's not spas or skincare labs—it's the food and beverage industry. Essential oils are used to flavor your food and to help preserve it. From fruit juice to chewing gum to meat, essential oils are all up in there. Orange oil is the number-one-selling essential oil globally because it's used in orange juice, perfume, household cleaners, *and* pesticides (orange oil is a major source for the limonene that powers lots of bug sprays that are safe enough to use in your house). Aromatherapy and spas only very recently started to take up even a sliver of the market. Think about it: When was the last time you had a session with an aromatherapist? But you've definitely smelled juice that was made more fragrant through the use of essential oils. You've definitely eaten canned foods that were made tastier with them. You've definitely tasted them in your soda.

Essential oils are all around us, even when we're not aware of their presence. Have you ever used massage oil? Soothed sore muscles with a scented Epsom salts bath? Used all-natural, DEET-free bug spray? All of these products contain essential oils. Even if you've never used any of these, I can promise you that essential oils can be found in a product sitting in your home right now. So the question is: At a time when most of us are hyperaware of every ingredient we ingest, apply, or spray . . . why don't we know anything about essential oils?

I have spent more time pondering this question than I would like to admit. As with all mysterious and wonderful things, there is no easy answer, but I have been able to identify one key issue: Essential oil product claims are vague and complicated. For example, you'll often find sneaky precursors like "thought to be" and "historically" and "anecdotally" prior to any health or efficacy claims about them, which naturally makes us suspicious.

There are a few reasons for this.

1. Essential oil regulation is super complicated.

In the United States, essential oils are regulated by the Food and Drug Administration (FDA), but those regulations vary according to use (i.e., cosmetic or drug). If the essential oil falls under the category of *cosmetic use*—something used to make us look prettier or smell better—then the regulations are relatively lax. As long as the product isn't contaminated or mislabeled and the manufacturer is deemed to be truthful and responsible about its marketing claims, no further scrutiny is applied. (Side note: The FDA isn't so great about keeping up with how many products are on the market or all of the claims companies make. So you should always be skeptical when reading cosmetic marketing claims unless a company provides some type of evidence to support them.)

But if the essential oil is marketed as a treatment or cure for a physical ailment or disease, then the FDA views the product as a *drug*. And the FDA is all over the drug industry. All drugs sold in the United States must be FDA-approved, and that approval process is intense—it requires many rounds of research, approvals, and clinical trials.

When it comes to the medicinal use of essential oils, manufacturers have to be extremely careful about their product claims. Some of the properties of specific essential oil compounds have been studied in depth and their effects are scientifically proved (we'll talk more about that later). But because there's a big difference between proving a benefit of an essential oil *component* and proving that this benefit applies to the essential oil *itself*, marketing language qualifiers like "thought to be" or "anecdotally" are often employed. They aren't meant to mislead you (let's hope), they're simply the result of companies acting in compliance with federal laws that are trying to keep you safe.

In the end, regulations intended to protect us from phony, harmful claims are the reason why it's so hard to prove the benefits of essential oils. So the claims you do see are couched in language that feels shaky and unconvincing. And because you're a smart person, you don't buy it, and you remain skeptical about essential oils.

Why isn't there some way to prove how awesome essential oils are? That is a fantastic question. And it's my next point!

2. Essential oils are difficult to study.

You may remember from high school chemistry class that all scientific evidence rests on establishing the relationship between cause and effect. For an experiment to be successful, it must prove a significant outcome that can be repeated over and over, and it must account for any variable that could affect the outcome. Does this ring a bell? To put it in terms that will make sense when it comes to beauty and drugs, an isolated component—an "active" ingredient—must be attributed to a certain effect; X ingredient must always produce Y result.

Imagine a hypothetical scenario where lab tests have shown that dropping a particular essential oil into a petri dish kills some type of virus. Sounds awesome, right? Sounds like proof? Well, unfortunately it's not. This is called "in vitro" testing, and it doesn't prove how something will work in the real world of the human body. There's still a looong way to go before a company could (or should!) claim that this essential oil is an effective drug for fighting the virus. First, study after study would need to be conducted to eliminate variables that might be playing into the oil's ability to kill the virus (was there something special about the way the lab technician handled the petri dish, or in the particular way the essential oil came into contact with the virus?). And second, researchers would have to identify the specific compounds of the oil responsible for killing the virus so that we could understand *exactly* how it worked.

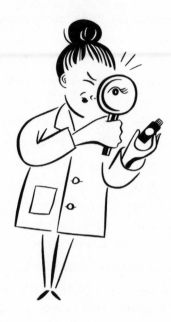

To control for all those variables would mean that scientists would need to make sure every batch of oils was identical and every compound was isolated (which, as we'll see in a bit, is close to impossible). And even if we could resolve those issues, we still wouldn't know for certain the effects of the oil *in an actual human body.* Would the active essential oil compounds survive long enough to kill the virus? Would there be too many side effects to make the drug worth it?

Of course, this is the standard applied to all drug testing. What makes it especially complicated when it comes to essential oils?

Well, first off, essential oils are made up of many complex parts; scientists are still trying to identify all of the different chemical compounds that appear in essential oils. And when researchers are able to isolate the compounds for testing, they end up with different results for each compound individually than when the oil is tested as a whole. This means that a whole essential oil is actually much more than the sum of its parts.

Additionally, because they are naturally occurring compounds and not synthetic chemicals created in a controlled environment, samples of essential oils can vary widely. This variability can be attributed to all kinds of factors. The way the crop was planted and harvested, what was in the soil, what the weather was like during the growing season, what weeds were present—all of this can impact the chemical composition of the finished essential oil.

Imagine trying to control for all of those variables in a clear, reliable, and repeatable study. No easy feat.

So whether you believe that our current way of regulating drugs is right or wrong, it definitely does not serve natural, complex ingredients well. At least right now, these regulatory standards make it tricky to explain the properties of essential oils through conventional research as we know it.

But that's not to say it can't be done. A lot of high-quality research exists that offers proof of the benefits of essential oils, and more is under way. Over the next couple of decades, our knowledge of essential oils is going to grow by leaps and bounds. That, to me, is one of the most exciting aspects of working with essential oils: It's only going to get better and better. Yes, it's going to take some time. Given that natural plant substances cannot easily be patented by companies, there is less profit potential and consequently less funding for research. But as consumers we have the power to affect that. The more we incorporate essential oils into our lives and the more we want to know about them, the more we'll help push the research forward.

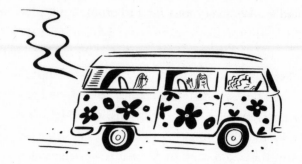

But for now, when you're standing in the health food store aisle wondering what to make of those little dark-glass vials, it can be frustrating not to have easy access to trustworthy information about them. You might turn to places like blogs or social media to find out what experts or friends are saying. There, you read things like, "Reverse the aging process with cinnamon oil!" and because you're a good critical thinker, you end up becoming skeptical about cinnamon oil. You roll your eyes and decide that whoever *does* believe that kind of non-sense probably drives around in a vintage Volkswagen camper, dances naked under the full moon, and reeks of patchouli oil. And that sucks because cinnamon oil actually *is* great. (And by the way, so is patchouli!)

3. Essential oil producers control a lot of the information available to the public.

You're going to learn a little bit about how essential oils are made in this book. At the end of it, you may even feel like you know enough to make them yourself. You probably won't, though. It's a complicated process that requires specific equipment, and it takes a very long time to produce a little bit of oil. It would require a ton of patience on your part, and the same is true for the companies that choose to manufacture and sell essential oils. They might have the equipment, but if they want to do it the correct and best possible way, they cannot speed up the process or make it less labor-intensive and less expensive.

I checked in with Daniel Alafetich, an engineer who builds essential oil distilleries and manufacturing equipment, about how complicated the process of making essential oils actually is. Here are a few of the eye-opening tidbits he offered:

- Depending on the plant, it can take from three to eight hours to fully distill its essential oil.
- Distilling an essential oil requires intense precision; too much water will make the oil acidic and not enough water will burn it. (I have smelled burned essential oil and I promise you, it is not pretty.)
- Many plants need to be distilled for their essential oils while they're still fresh—as they dry, the oil vanishes.
- Contamination with plants other than the one you want (like weeds in the field, for instance) will change the composition of an oil.

As you can see, it's not easy to extract essential oils from plants. Very, very few companies have figured out how to make high-quality essential oils. And they aren't exactly open to sharing the information they learn along the way.

Of course, as with the research, these processes are also evolving. New suppliers are popping up on the market every day, and many of them have passion and integrity. I trust that eventually we'll have tons of options. Until then, the people who produce the goods also hold the keys to a huge vault of . . . secrets. That's essentially what they are: trade secrets. You and I don't get to know everything that they know. What we get instead is marketing claims—carefully manicured information meant to help sell the product, not necessarily to tell the whole truth.

Not to worry, though. I've spent years investigating essential oils, and I'm here to crack the case. I put a lot (a lot) of work into finding suppliers, aromatherapists, experts, and even some skeptics that I trust, and I tapped them all (like trees) for information. I've also diffused and experimented and DIYed with more oils than I can count. In the coming chapters, I will share everything I've learned . . . and (aside from this amazing book, thankyouverymuch) I'm not going to try to sell you anything.

A NOTE ON DIRECT-SALES MODELS

A direct-sales model (aka a multilevel marketing company) is one in which "regular" people—think your neighbor, sister, or mom—sell products on behalf of a large company directly to their network. While a lot of younger people these days have never come in contact with direct-sales models (I'm in my thirties and they're new to me!), they've been around a long time and are actually common and thriving. Maybe you know about Avon or Mary Kay, both of which are pioneers in the beauty industry and still going strong. (Avon was founded in 1886 and made $10 billion in 2013!) In a direct-sales model, the salespeople or members get paid through product, product discounts, and commission every time someone buys products directly from them. In some versions of the sales model, members can bring in another salesperson under them, and get commission through that person's sales.

A lot of people are suspicious of direct selling, but I do think it has its benefits. A few decades ago, especially, it offered women a way to work from home and make their own money. As a small-business owner, I'm also super into the idea of cutting out the retailer middleman and selling our products straight to our community. It's a cliché but it's true: Word of mouth is the best marketing there is.

The problem is that sometimes these companies hide behind their salespeople and let them make claims on behalf of the company itself, slowing down regulators' ability to stop false or misleading claims. Salespeople whose entire training came from the brand they're representing should not be trusted when they claim that their product "cures Ebola" (yes, this has really happened). They are not qualified to make therapeutic claims about the product, and they are making money every time they convince you to buy it. This should at the very least concern you and, in my opinion, make you want to walk away and shop elsewhere.

Direct-sales models are incredibly common in the essential oil industry, and the companies that employ them are huge. Some have received warning letters from the FDA about their business practices, yet they continue to grow and dominate the market. I encourage you to do your research and be a skeptic. If what you read really convinces you, that's wonderful. Maybe you feel there is more than enough evidence that the product is right for you. Just always remember that marketing is marketing, no matter who it comes from.

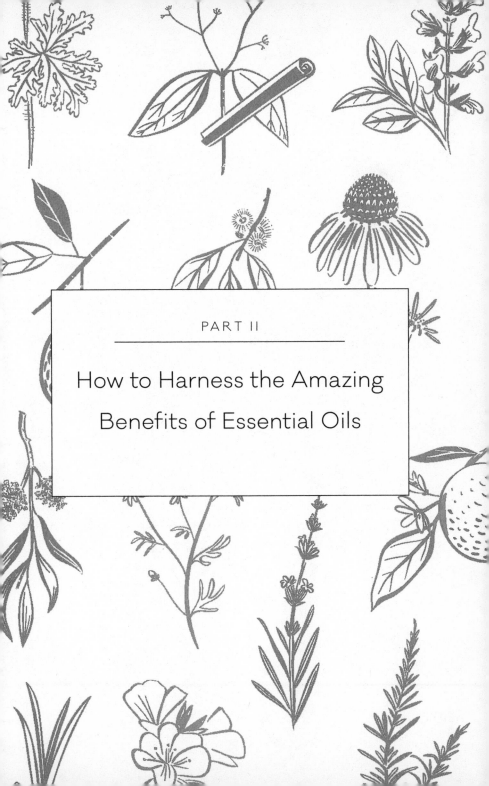

PART II

How to Harness the Amazing Benefits of Essential Oils

CHAPTER 4

Essential Oils Stripped Down

We know that essential oils are powerful plant substances and that their molecular complexity makes them tricky for scientists to study. But what *are* these magical components that fuel plant life and enhance human life? And what exactly can they *do* for us?

I want to take a moment to talk about the components of essential oils because, as with anything else, the more you understand about their properties, the better able you will be to incorporate them into your life in helpful ways. Each component of an essential oil offers its own host of benefits; in fact, manufacturers of beauty products inject isolated plant compounds into their products to make them more effective.

"cold-pressed," "raw," and "unrefined." Even if you end up ordering them online once you get into your groove, I recommend doing some in-person research before you buy for the first time. Check out the oils at your neighborhood natural grocery store or holistic beauty shop and get a sense of the different levels of quality available. It won't take you much time to notice the difference between a fiber-filled, vibrant olive oil and one that looks like Vitaminwater.

Here are some of my favorite carrier oils.

Olive Oil

If you read *Skin Cleanse*, you know that olive oil is a skin-care ingredient that I consider to be essential. It's also highly underrated. For one, it's extremely affordable and is so easy to find that you probably only have to walk into your kitchen to get it. Moreover, it's so, so good for your skin. It protects it from sun damage, offers anti-aging benefits, and is very gentle. And while everyone's skin is different, I have encountered very few people who have a sensitivity to olive oil.

Sweet Almond Oil

Sweet almond oil is a staple ingredient in the S.W. Basics product line and in lots of other natural brands because, like olive oil, it helps heal the skin from sun damage and can reverse the signs of aging. It also helps to even out your skin tone and fight inflammation, which makes it great for distressed and irritated skin. Plus, it's gentle and light, meaning it's a fairly unobtrusive carrier oil.

Avocado Oil

We all know how beneficial avocados are, so it's not hard to imagine that pressing all of those supernutrients into an oil would do wonders for your health. Avocado oil is a thick, lush oil that is high in antioxidants and omega-3 fatty acids *and* full of vitamins and minerals. When it comes to skincare, it contains natural steroids that may help your skin to produce more collagen, plus it's super-duper moisturizing. I like to use it in recipes that are formulated to heal damaged skin or dry hair. (PS: Feel free to rub avocados straight onto your skin . . . that works too!)

Jojoba Oil

Jojoba oil it is actually not an oil but a liquid wax. This gives it a *five-year* shelf life that far exceeds most other carrier oils. Jojoba oil makes a great choice for a carrier oil because it is an almost perfect match, chemically, to your skin's sebum (the oil it produces to protect itself), which means that it is easily absorbed. Jojoba oil also has antibacterial and antifungal properties.

CHOOSING THE RIGHT JOJOBA

The quality of jojoba oil varies a lot depending on the sourcing method and brand. At S.W. Basics we get our jojoba oil from Oro de Sonora, a family-owned and -operated certified organic farm and processor. When I first tried their oil, I was a total beginner. I wrote to Allie Aronstam, who's in charge of selling to companies like mine, saying her oil smelled funny. She graciously schooled me, teaching me about the realities of refined oils (which have no smell). So I've asked her to school all of us here on how to choose a quality jojoba oil. Her guidelines can also be applied in a more general sense when it comes to choosing any carrier oil. Keep in mind that even though she's specifically referring to jojoba oil, these rules apply to all carrier oils.

"First off, jojoba should have a nutty, slightly earthy odor. If you purchase jojoba oil that has no scent at all, it most likely has been deodorized."

"Second, jojoba should be golden and viscous. If you purchase a jojoba oil that is clear or very light yellow, with a lightweight feeling, you probably have a refined jojoba oil. Refined jojoba is never a high-quality jojoba—the refining process strips away all of its important properties."

"Not only do some jojoba oils undergo deodorizing and refining processes, but certain manufacturers also use hexane solvents to extract the oil. When jojoba oil is first pressed with an expeller it is about 40–45 percent oil and 55–60 percent leftover meal. That meal still contains some of the liquid wax esters. This is where a secondary process called solvent extraction comes in. The jojoba meal is washed in a hexane solution and then heated to a temperature that allows for the hexane to vaporize, leaving you with a usable jojoba oil. This oil is sometimes blended with first press oil in order for processors to get the most value out of their seeds. When purchasing jojoba, always opt for a first press over a blended oil."

Rosehip Seed Oil

Rosehip seed oil, which is harvested from the seeds of rosebushes, is a little bit more obscure than the other oils on this list. But I'm including it here because I think it makes an excellent carrier oil, particularly when it comes to skincare. It's incredibly light and delicate, meaning it absorbs into the skin quickly without leaving behind a greasy residue, and it contains high levels of skin-friendly essential fatty acids. I've found that it works well for mature and acne-prone skin alike.

Coconut Oil

Unlike rosehip seed oil, coconut oil is well known. I'm sure you've read a trillion things about its benefits in the past few years. It has grown rapidly in popularity in both healthy food and skincare circles for good reason: It's amazing. Loaded with healthy fats and antioxidants, coconut oil is incredibly nourishing. It also has antibacterial and antifungal properties, which make it a great addition to germ-killing products like toothpaste and mouthwash. (Recipes for both coming up soon, obvs!)

Evening Primrose Oil

Primrose oil is a light, easily absorbed oil that's high in omega-6 fatty acids. It helps to alleviate the symptoms of eczema and dermatitis, and it may even help with balancing hormones. It is sold as a supplement to take internally, but I also recommend it as a carrier oil for very sensitive skin. If you're prone to dry, itchy skin or struggle with skin conditions or rashes, this one is for you!

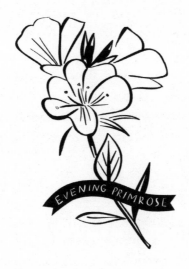

Sesame Oil

Sesame oil is derived from—you guessed it—sesame seeds. Fairly lightweight and possessing a nice, nutty aroma, it's a versatile carrier oil (make sure you're getting untoasted sesame unless you want to smell like Chinese food). Like coconut oil and jojoba oil it offers antibacterial and anti-fungal benefits, plus it's antiviral and anti-inflammatory. Just be aware that, although this is rare with most skincare ingredients, a dietary allergy to sesame will also result in an intolerance for topical application.

DILUTION GUIDELINES

All the recipes in this book call for a carrier oil or water-based solution to dilute the potency of the essential oil. For most of these recipes, I've offered a range for dilution. If you are extremely sensitive to new products and ingredients, start at the low end of the range. If your skin is tough or you have a lot of experience using essential oils, go for the higher amount (that's what I do, but I worked my way up to it!). Dilution ratios vary quite a bit depending on the essential oil, but here are a few general guidelines to keep in mind:

- In skin treatments (massage oils, scrubs, lotions, creams), 1 tablespoon of a carrier oil will support 6–15 drops of a given essential oil.
- For products you are applying to your face, exercise more caution. I'd recommend 1 tablespoon of a carrier oil to support 3–7 drops of a given essential oil.
- For a bath, use 2–12 drops total. While some sources say you can add the drops directly into the water, I recommend mixing the essential oil into an oil, salt, or sugar first. Otherwise the essential oil will sit on top of the bathwater and can hit your skin all at once. Intense!
- For your diffuser, follow the dilution instructions in the manual that comes with it.
- For steam inhalation, use 3–7 drops total at a time, adding drops as they evaporate.
- For a room or cleaning spray, use 10–20 drops per tablespoon of liquid.

Each of the recipes that follow has been tested and tailored according to its specific ingredients. You'll see some variation in quantities from formula to formula. Besides testing essential oils on a patch of skin before using them in a recipe, I also suggest testing each skincare recipe on a patch of skin (ideally your hand or your inner arm) before putting it on your face or all over your body.

Okay, enough with the warnings. It's time to *have fun*!

SKINCARE

Sales in the global skincare market exceed $121 billion annually. Can you believe that? And it's growing every day. The great news is that while more products are available than ever before, consumers are also more educated than ever before and are becoming more and more selective about their purchases. Natural and organic products are on the rise, and many stores are doing away with pushy salespeople who don't offer customers real information. This all makes me so happy. But the thing that makes me the happiest is when I meet people (more and more of them each day) who tell me that they're making their own skincare products. Because making your own skincare products is the best way to learn about your body and, specifically, your skin. It allows you to fully control the ingredients that come into contact with your face and body and makes shopping for products that much easier—you'll know which ingredients to seek out and which ones to avoid.

The recipes that follow are designed to highlight essential oils in ways that benefit your skin. Pay close attention to how your skin responds. Sometimes you will experience a few breakouts as part of the cleansing/detox process, but this should never last longer than a couple of days. Take it slowly—you do not need to make and use all of these recipes in one day. Test out one at a time and give them some room to work!

Breakout Clearing Cleanser

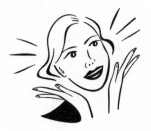

Featuring three of the most potent acne-fighting essential oils—clary sage, lavender, and tea tree oil—this cleanser will become your new go-to when you're feeling a breakout coming on. Unlike many acne face washes, this cleanser won't make your skin feel supertight and dry afterward. You can thank lavender's anti-inflammatory and hydrating properties for that, as well as the vegetable glycerin, which will help moisturize your skin as you wash it.

¼ cup lavender hydrosol
¼ cup vegetable glycerin
3–9 drops clary sage essential oil
2–6 drops tea tree essential oil

Combine lavender hydrosol and vegetable glycerin in a small pot and bring to a boil. Allow to cool, then pour into a 4-ounce glass bottle. Add essential oils and shake well before using. Use a coin-sized amount on wet or dry skin, rubbing in circular motions. Rinse off with water thoroughly. This product will last up to 1 year and will make about 20 uses.

MAKE YOUR OWN HYDROSOL!

Adrienne Ahnell, our source for lavender hydrosol, taught me how to make an amazing stovetop hydrosol. This is a great way to spend less money and to ensure your hydrosol is *real*, and not watered down with other ingredients.

1. Put 4–5 handfuls of dried rose petals or lavender buds in a large pot.
2. Add 6 cups of distilled water.
3. Mix the liquid with clean hands, swirling the petals around. This might turn the water pink!
4. Place a small ceramic bowl facedown in the pot as a base and another wide-mouth bowl faceup on top of it as the collection bowl. Make sure it is balanced and that the bowls you use are heat resistant.
5. Place a lid on the pot upside down so it curves toward the bottom. That way, when the steam from the rose petals hits the top of the lid, it will funnel down into the collection bowl. Place a bag of ice cubes, tightly sealed, on top of the concave, upside-down lid. Heat the liquid to a boil and immediately turn it down to medium to simmer.
6. Set a timer to 20 minutes. Steam will rise to the top and condense when it hits the cold top and drip down into the collection bowl. After 20 minutes, the hydrosol is ready. Pour it into a jar and put in the fridge.

The hydrosol should be superclear, unlike the red rose tea at the bottom of the pot. Makes about ½ cup of liquid; use within 6 months.

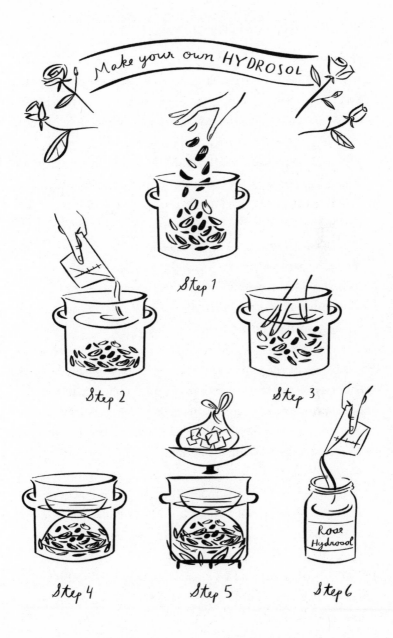

Make your own HYDROSOL

Step 1

Step 2

Step 3

Step 4

Step 5

Step 6

Rose Hydrosol

The Ultimate Oil Cleanser

Oil cleansing is all the rage these days. Avocado oil and rose-hip seed oil are both light oils that are supernutrient-dense. They'll help clear up clogged pores, whiteheads, and blackheads while providing deep hydration. Carrot seed oil will tone oily skin, plus will assist in smoothing out fine lines and wrinkles. Bergamot oil will balance the strong scent of carrot seed and kill bacteria on the skin. This is a good one if you deal with oily skin and clogged pores. You'll definitely feel it working!

1 tablespoon avocado oil
1 tablespoon rosehip seed oil
5–10 drops carrot seed essential oil
4–8 drops bergamot essential oil

Combine all of the ingredients and store in a 1-ounce sealed glass bottle or tightly covered glass bowl. Use a quarter-sized amount on wet or dry skin, rubbing in circular motions. Follow with a soapy face wash. You can store this product for up to 1 year, and it will make about 24 uses.

Warm 'n' Cozy Mask

The combination of myrrh, tangerine, and clove oil in this mask results in a wonderful, warm, uplifting aroma that makes me feel like curling up in an adult onesie. Scent aside, these also happen to be deeply healing and restorative skin oils. Lactic acid–rich yogurt helps to exfoliate dead skin cells, moisturize, and even out your skin tone. The exfoliation is a bit intense, so add the optional carrier oil if you have super-sensitive skin.

3 tablespoons plain full-fat Greek yogurt
2 drops myrrh essential oil
2 drops tangerine essential oil
1 drop clove essential oil
OPTIONAL: *1 tablespoon carrier oil*

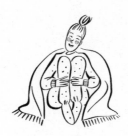

Combine all of the ingredients in a glass bowl. Apply a quarter-sized amount all over your face, beginning at the center and working your way outward to your hairline and jawline. Apply more if needed until your skin is completely covered. Leave on until dry and rinse off thoroughly. Store covered in the fridge, but use within a week because the oils will evaporate from the mixture. Makes 2 or 3 uses.

Teatime Oily Skin Mask

This mask is great for you extra-oily, breakout-prone folks out there. French green clay is one of the most powerful pore-clearing ingredients I've encountered: I swear you can literally feel it pulling the toxins out of your skin. Don't be scared, though, because I've cut some of its potency by pairing it with supersoothing, antibacterial honey and soothing olive oil. Studies have shown that those deficient in linoleic acid are more likely to suffer from acne. Cheers! Or . . . whatever you say when you're toasting at a tea party.

1 tablespoon olive oil
1 tablespoon honey
1 tablespoon French green clay
1 teaspoon water
4 drops bergamot essential oil
2 drops chamomile essential oil

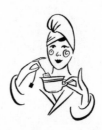

Combine all of the ingredients in a glass bowl. Apply a quarter-sized amount all over your face, beginning at the center and working your way outward to your hairline and jawline. Leave on until dry and then rinse off thoroughly. Makes 1 use.

Florida Face Scrub

This colorful, beautiful scrub combines some of my favorite things into one potent exfoliator. Oat flour will gently remove dead skin cells, while the avocado *and* carrier oil provide hydration in the form of skin-saving omega fatty acids. (Plus you can use up that soft avocado you let sit out for too long.) The grapefruit and sweet orange add some nice light scent, plus help target acne and alleviate oil imbalances. This scrub is supersoothing to sensitive skin.

2 tablespoons oat flour
½ ripe avocado, mashed
2 teaspoons carrier oil
2 drops sweet orange essential oil
2 drops grapefruit essential oil

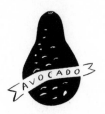

Combine all of the ingredients in a glass bowl. Use a generous amount and apply all over your face, beginning at the center and working your way outward to your hairline and jawline. Apply more if needed until your skin is completely covered. Feel free to use this on your whole body, otherwise it will make 2 uses for your face. The avocado will not keep, though, so share any excess or toss it.

Super Luxe Floral Face Toner

This is a toner for when you really want to treat yourself and feel like Kate Middleton or Beyoncé (America's Kate). The rosewater base helps to hydrate your skin, even out discoloration, and reduce redness. Rose otto essential oil is wonderful for mature, dry, or sensitive skin and pairs gorgeously with the equally aromatic jasmine essential oil (which can help with acne and inflammation). All hail, queen.

¼ cup rosewater
4–12 drops rose otto essential oil
2–6 drops jasmine essential oil

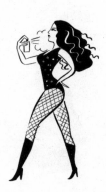

Combine all of the ingredients in a glass bowl. Apply to your face with a cotton ball or cloth or, if you have a 2-ounce glass spritz bottle, transfer the toner to the bottle and lightly spritz onto your face. Do not rinse. Rose otto and jasmine usually come diluted into carrier oil, which will shorten the shelf life, so store this toner in an airtight container for up to 3 months. Makes at least 60 uses.

Sweet-and-Spicy Body Scrub

This is a riff on the S.W. Basics body scrub, but a bit more racy. Coarse sugar will naturally exfoliate and soften your bod, while the carrier oil provides hydration. Nutmeg and ginger are a spicy, bright combination that helps to soothe inflammation, increase circulation, ease body aches and pains, and relieve stress.

1 cup organic coarse sugar
1 tablespoon carrier oil
10–20 drops nutmeg essential oil
5–10 drops ginger essential oil

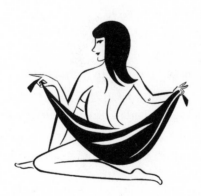

Combine all of the ingredients in a glass bowl. Scoop a generous handful and apply using circulation motions to wet arms, legs, back, or stomach. Rinse thoroughly. Store scrub in an airtight container for up to 6 months. (Be sure to keep it somewhere other than the edge of the bathtub—if water seeps in it will spoil quickly.) Makes about 12 uses.

Moisturizing Spot Treatment

I know the title of this one sounds like an oxymoron, but believe it or not, one of the reasons your skin breaks out is that it's *dry*. In response to the dryness, it overproduces oil, and that excess oil makes you break out. This treatment will balance oil production and kill bacteria. I whipped it up while on a business trip with ingredients I found at Target, and it took me five minutes to make. So you have no excuse. (I like to use it over my entire face, but it makes a great spot treatment.)

1 tablespoon argan oil
1 tablespoon grapeseed oil
30 drops lavender essential oil
10 drops peppermint essential oil
5–10 drops eucalyptus essential oil

Combine all of the ingredients in a glass bottle, preferably with a dropper. Using a cotton ball or your hands, apply a very small amount of the treatment directly to the offending culprit. Leave on for as long as you can (I recommend applying before bed). Store treatment in an airtight container for up to 1 year. Makes about 30 uses.

Marvin Gaye Massage Oil

Ylang ylang and neroli oils are both renowned for their aph-rodisiac and libido-enhancing qualities, hence their presence in this sultry massage oil. I think you'll love the slightly sweet, fresh aroma of the two combined—plus they're antispasmodic, antidepressant, and anti-inflammatory. Coconut oil is a very lush carrier oil with a wonderful sweet scent, while adding another carrier oil helps make the whole combination glide on supersmooth. Wink, wink.

¼ cup coconut oil
¼ cup carrier oil
10–20 drops ylang ylang essential oil
5–10 drops neroli essential oil

Combine all of the ingredients in a glass bowl or bottle. Use a liberal amount all over your body, applying in wide, circular motions. Store any remaining massage oil in an airtight con-tainer for up to 6 months. Makes several uses . . . or just 1. De-pends on how your night goes. (Word of caution: This recipe is meant to be pregame and is not safe as a lubricant, especially with condoms! #practicesafesex.)

PERFUME

The following recipes feature a simple formula for perfume that even the most DIY-adverse will have no problem acing. For each of them, you'll need 1 tablespoon of at least 100-proof alcohol (190-proof is best, because it's odorless; you can grab Everclear from the liquor store you frequent), and 1½ teaspoons of distilled water, which you can buy at any grocery store. You can replace the alcohol and water with jojoba oil, but bear in mind that this will shorten your perfume's shelf life, alter its scent, and reduce the amount of time it lingers on your skin.

One very important thing to keep in mind: *Your water must be distilled.* Tap water is not acceptable here, because of the potential for bacterial growth. As with any natural product that contains water, mold can still happen, so be sure to periodically check your perfume for signs of cloudiness or growth.

For each recipe, I recommend using between 30 and 45 drops of essential oil. Don't add them haphazardly: You should add them in a precise order that corresponds to their designation as the base, middle, or top notes of your fragrance. No idea what base, middle, and top notes are? Let me explain.

You know how an aroma kind of changes from the time you first apply it? If you spray on a perfume in the morning, chances are it will smell totally different by the time you come home from work at night. This phenomenon can largely be explained by the concept of fragrance "notes." The top note is the aroma you smell first—it also happens to be the fastest evaporating. The middle note is the scent you'll smell next, and the base note is the slowest-evaporating, longest-lingering smell. So, yes, your fragrance will change as time goes on because the various layers of fragrance ("notes") are evaporating from your skin at different times. Making perfume is really an art form.

Here's an overview of the basic process for making perfume:

- Begin by mixing together the alcohol and the distilled water in a glass bottle. Next, add your essential oils. Create your blend a drop at a time, smelling as you go (remember you can always add more of an oil but you can never subtract).
- Begin with your base notes and then proceed to your middle notes and top notes.
- Shake the whole combination together and store, tightly covered, in a cool, dark place. The perfume can be stored from 48 hours to 6 weeks—it all depends on how potent you want your fragrance to be (the longer it sits, the stronger it will be).
- Once it's reached the scent you desire, decant your mixture into a spritz bottle or a bottle with a roller top and, again, shake vigorously. You're ready! Your perfume should keep for at least a year, if not longer.

The Scent Rainbow

It's really tempting to categorize fragrances as "masculine" or "feminine," but gender norms are so passé. Perfumers break scents into all kinds of nuanced categories (some with crazy names like "chypre fruity" and "oriental fougere"). We don't need to go into that kind of detail, but the chart below will give you a general idea of how you can think through different scents when you're blending your own perfumes.

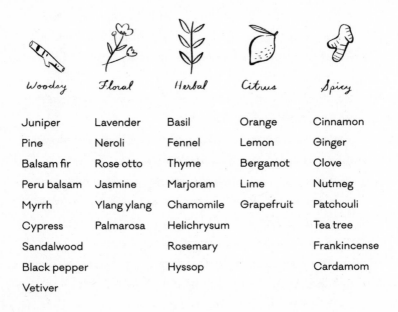

Woodsy	Floral	Herbal	Citrus	Spicy
Juniper	Lavender	Basil	Orange	Cinnamon
Pine	Neroli	Fennel	Lemon	Ginger
Balsam fir	Rose otto	Thyme	Bergamot	Clove
Peru balsam	Jasmine	Marjoram	Lime	Nutmeg
Myrrh	Ylang ylang	Chamomile	Grapefruit	Patchouli
Cypress	Palmarosa	Helichrysum		Tea tree
Sandalwood		Rosemary		Frankincense
Black pepper		Hyssop		Cardamom
Vetiver				

Sexy Sandalwood Perfume

Sandalwood is one of those aromas that I just don't seem to tire of: It's sexy, smoky, earthy, and warm. Cedarwood is similar in scent and enhances those qualities, while palmarosa and rose otto offer a bit of a welcome contrast—they're sweet, bright, and floral. Wear this before a big date or anytime you're feeling down with your bad self.

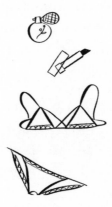

1 tablespoon alcohol
1½ teaspoons distilled water
BASE NOTE: 18 drops sandalwood essential oil
MIDDLE NOTE: 6 drops cedarwood essential oil
TOP NOTE: 8 drops palmarosa essential oil or rose otto
  essential oil

Julia's Perfume

This perfume is inspired by my friend Julia's favorite "conventional" fragrance, Florence by the perfumery Tocca. Now, Julia also happens to work with me here at S.W. Basics and, as with all my employees, my product sensitivity rubbed off on her. Sadly—or luckily, really—she can no longer tolerate synthetic perfume of any kind. This fragrance riffs on the musky-sweet-citrusy combination that she loves, but won't cause her to break out in hives. It's a fantastic blend for anyone who likes floral scents but doesn't want something too sickly sweet.

1 tablespoon alcohol
1½ teaspoons distilled water
BASE NOTE: *12 drops bergamot essential oil*
MIDDLE NOTE: *12 drops jasmine essential oil*
TOP NOTE: *6 drops grapefruit essential oil*

"Dude" Perfume

I'm refusing to call this cologne, even though most men's perfumes are designated as such (please also take those quotes to mean that this fragrance isn't just for men, but it's classically "masculine"). If you've smelled a men's cologne before, chances are you've smelled something laced with vetiver. It's a common base note, renowned for its spicy, woodsy aroma. Here, I've paired it with equally woodsy patchouli, plus sweet orange, which is a quintessential top note for thicker, warmer fragrances. FYI, I would totally wear this scent.

1 tablespoon alcohol
1½ teaspoons distilled water
BASE NOTE: *15 drops vetiver essential oil*
MIDDLE NOTE: *10 drops patchouli essential oil*
TOP NOTE: *10 drops sweet orange essential oil*

Pharaoh Perfume

This blend is inspired by the Ancient Egyptians' love of fragrance. And this blend truly encapsulates the scents of the time. Myrrh and frankincense are both ancient essential oils—perhaps the oldest documented ones in history—and were heavily favored by Egyptian pharaohs as scents of the gods. The lotus flower was a sacred and holy plant in Ancient Egypt and, today, its essential oil remains hard to procure and expensive. Rose absolute is a nice substitute, offering a similarly heady, indulgent aroma that is a nice top note.

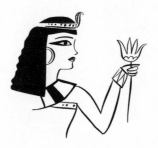

1 tablespoon alcohol
1½ teaspoons distilled water
BASE NOTE: *10 drops myrrh essential oil*
MIDDLE NOTE: *10 drops frankincense essential oil*
TOP NOTE: *10 drops white lotus absolute or rose absolute essential oil*

Florescent Perfume

Susannah Compton is the founder and formulator of Florescent, a line of handcrafted perfumes made from organic essential oils and absolutes. She taught me how to make perfume (the right way) and shares a perfume with us here:

"If you crave chocolate as much as I do, this delectable perfume will allow you to indulge your senses without the sugar crash. Cacao absolute lends the warm and cozy aroma of fine dark chocolate. Rose absolute is the quintessential tonic of the heart, and it enhances your capacity for love—for both yourself and others. Rose truly elevates the cacao absolute. I mean, when do roses and chocolate *not* go together? Pink peppercorn adds intrigue and lift with its slightly floral, warm, and dry spice appeal."

1 tablespoon alcohol
1½ teaspoons distilled water
BASE NOTE: *15 drops cacao absolute*
MIDDLE NOTE: *10 drops rose absolute*
TOP NOTE: *5 drops pink peppercorn essential oil*

One and Done

If you're low-key like me (aka *lazy*), here is a recipe using sexy-smelling oils that make great perfumes all by themselves. No need to worry about top, middle, or base notes here—just add 30 drops of whichever essential oil you love the most and use in the same way you would any of the other perfumes above!

2 tablespoons alcohol
1 tablespoon distilled water
30 drops Peru balsam, palmarosa, patchouli, rose otto,
*   sandalwood, ylang ylang, jasmine, or neroli essential oil*

BLENDS FROM THE EXPERTS

SUSAN GRIFFIN-BLACK

Susan Griffin-Black is a pioneer in the essential oils space and an expert in aromatherapy and the chemistry of perfumery. She cofounded EO Products in 1995. EO stands for essential oils, and the aromatic essences of plants are the heart and soul of every product they produce. Susan is a true alchemist with essential oils, and EO's blends are some of the best-smelling products I've ever come across, period. Here, she shares with us three quick blends you can make easily at home.

Healing Blend

Helichrysum, also known as immortelle, is a lesser-known essential oil. Emotionally, helichrysum is good for all sorts of broken-heart healing. Physically, it's great for healing injuries to the skin—it helps to regenerate collagen and can be applied to bumps and bruises on skin to accelerate healing. Use this blend in a diffuser or as a room spray—just transfer to a spray bottle and add 8 ounces of distilled water.

2 tablespoons carrier oil (such as sweet almond)
6 drops helichrysum essential oil
8 drops lavender essential oil
2 drops palmarosa essential oil
2 drops lemon essential oil

   Mix all of the ingredients in a small glass jar and store in a cool, dark place. Makes 1 use in a diffuser (skip the carrier oil) and more than 60 uses as a room spray. Will last up to 2 years.

Grounding Blend

Palmarosa is a grassy, earthy, rosy-sweet essential oil that makes a lovely middle note for fragrances. Sweet orange oil is uplifting, balancing, and known for its antibacterial properties. Blend with lavender and use this elixir as a restorative bath oil or in a room diffuser.

2 tablespoons carrier oil (if using in a bath)
6 drops palmarosa essential oil
9 drops lavender essential oil
3 drops sweet orange essential oil

Combine the essential oils without the carrier oil in a diffuser for 1 use. For a bath oil, combine all of the ingredients in a bottle and shake well, pouring out half into a bath. Makes 2 uses and will last up to 1 year.

Find Your Balance Blend

Rose geranium is one of my favorite essences in smell, feel, and its ability to bring balance to any situation. It's even said to be good for balancing female hormones. When it's blended with sweet orange and rose absolute essential oils, the synergy is simply magical. Use as aromatherapy or a bath oil—just add a few drops to the water and enjoy the relaxing steam.

2 tablespoons carrier oil (jojoba is my favorite)
9 drops rose geranium essential oil
6 drops sweet orange essential oil
3 drops rose absolute essential oil

Mix all of the ingredients in a small glass jar and apply to pulse points. Store in a cool dark place for up to 2 years. Makes 2 bath uses or 2 years of sniffs as aromatherapy.

PERSONAL CARE

While some of us can get away with not using that much skincare (like yours truly, who is basically on a permanent skin cleanse), personal care is unavoidable. It is a constant part of our daily lives, from our hair to our teeth to our pits. Think about how often you put on deodorant. Don't you want that product to be clean and good for your health? Me too. What about the toothpaste or mouthwash you accidentally swallow sometimes? Or the shampoo that runs down your entire body?

To me, personal-care products should be the gentlest of them all. Enter the superheroes below. They'll take good care of you, I promise.

Rosemary Clarifying Shampoo

The problem with many clarifying shampoos is that they are really, really harsh on your scalp. This recipe not only will remove buildup but will help treat dry, distressed skin—which, honestly, is often the root cause of hair dullness. Rosemary acts like a tonic for the scalp, alleviating dandruff and increasing circulation. Apple cider vinegar will help clear up product accumulation and leave your hair extra shiny and conditioned, while the carrier oil will ensure your hair doesn't get too dried out.

¼ cup unscented castile liquid soap (like Dr. Bronner's)
1 teaspoon apple cider vinegar
1 teaspoon carrier oil
3–6 drops rosemary essential oil

Combine all of the ingredients in a bowl and then transfer to an 8-ounce glass bottle. Shake well before use. Apply as you would with your normal shampoo and rinse thoroughly. Store for up to 1 month; will make at least 15 uses.

Choco-Mint Dry Shampoo

Ah, dry shampoo: the lazy person's cheat for good hair. Sometimes it takes a *lot* of work to rub it all in thoroughly. Since we can't all be blondes (or bottle blondes), this recipe integrates cocoa powder to help "dye" the mixture to more accurately fit your hair shade. Have fun experimenting with the right ratio of cocoa powder to arrowroot powder/cornstarch, but try to keep it to around 4 tablespoons total. As for the peppermint essential oil: It adds a refreshing aroma, plus will help soothe dry and itchy scalps. This dry shampoo works amazingly, and, I gotta say, it's pretty nice to smell like a mint chocolate bar all day!

FOR BLOND/WHITE HAIR:
4 tablespoons arrowroot powder or cornstarch

FOR LIGHT BROWN HAIR:
3 tablespoons arrowroot powder or cornstarch
1 tablespoon cocoa powder

FOR BROWN/BLACK HAIR:
2 tablespoons arrowroot powder or cornstarch
2 tablespoons cocoa powder

THEN, FOR ALL HAIR COLORS:
Add 7 drops peppermint essential oil

Combine all of the ingredients in a bowl and then transfer to a small glass jar. Sprinkle as much or little as necessary directly onto your scalp, using circular motions to rub it in. (Really dig in there, so the peppermint has a chance to work its magic.) This can be a bit messy while you're using it, so I usually step in the tub and apply it before getting dressed. Store in an airtight container for up to 2 years, though you may need to refresh the peppermint oil as it loses potency. Number of uses will vary depending on how oily your hair is, but you should get at least 12 uses out of this recipe.

Nighttime Dandruff Treatment

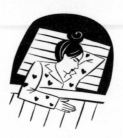

I recommend using this treatment at night for two reasons: One, you can let it really sink in and work. Two, you *might* look a little greasy after you apply it. Fear not. Jojoba oil is both light and nourishing; applying it directly on your scalp will immediately alleviate dryness and irritation. Plus, the dandruff-busting, bacteria-killing, and skin-soothing trifecta of lemongrass, lavender, and tea tree essential oils is nothing short of miraculous. It's really, really worth the temporarily greasy hair.

1 tablespoon jojoba oil
3–6 drops lemongrass essential oil
2–4 drops lavender essential oil
1–2 drops tea tree essential oil

Combine all of the ingredients in a bowl and then transfer to a small bottle. Apply directly to your scalp with your fingers, rubbing in using circular motions. Leave on overnight. Shower and shampoo in the morning. Store in an airtight container for up to 1 year. Makes 2–3 uses.

Rose Chamomile Conditioning Rinse

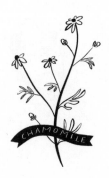

Cooled chamomile tea is one of my favorite natural ingredients, as it helps brighten up hair and, if you're a blonde, can actually enhance the color. The base of this recipe pairs chamomile with gentle, ultra-moisturizing aloe juice. (If your hair is feeling extra dry, add in the optional carrier oil—argan oil is a good choice.) The chamomile and rose otto essential oils are both soothing, anxiety-relieving oils that are great for treating fragile and damaged hair. Plus, they smell wondrous.

¼ cup aloe juice, powder, or the inside of a fresh aloe leaf
¼ cup cooled chamomile tea
3–7 drops chamomile essential oil
3–7 drops rose otto essential oil
1 teaspoon carrier oil (optional, for extra hydration)

Combine all of the ingredients in a bowl. Apply to wet hair after shampooing and either rinse as you would a normal conditioner or leave on for up to 20 minutes, then rinse thoroughly. This recipe should make 1 use.

Non-Greasy Beard Oil

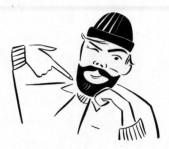

Perhaps the most common complaint I hear about beard oils is that they leave the beard oily and sticky, not soft and groomed. This recipe's base is rosehip seed oil, which is light and fast absorbing, so your beard—or your man's beard—will be nourished but *not* greasy. Thyme linalool (also known as sweet thyme) essential oil is a potent antimicrobial agent; while it's great for addressing underlying conditions like acne, it is still gentle enough to be used, diluted, on the skin. The addition of Roman chamomile provides a nice sweet citrus aroma, plus it is a wonderful, calming oil that can be used to alleviate the symptoms of irritated skin.

2 tablespoons rosehip seed oil
2–5 drops thyme linalool essential oil
4–7 drops Roman chamomile essential oil

Combine all of the ingredients in a glass bottle (I recommend using one that can fit a dropper top). Shake thoroughly before use. Use a dime-sized amount and apply thoroughly, using your fingertips. Store in a cool, dark place for up to 1 year. Makes 12 uses depending on the size of your beard, you stud you.

Woodsy Witch Hazel Aftershave

Shaving through ingrown hairs and inflamed pores is a universal concern for men and women, but some of the most distressed, damaged skin I've seen is a man's face after shaving: It's raw, red, and supersensitive. The witch hazel in this aftershave will alleviate inflammation and kill bacteria, while the carrier oil will hydrate irritated skin. Aside from lending it a woodsy aroma, the cypress and sandalwood essential oils assist in treating acne, improving circulation, and toning oily skin.

2 tablespoons witch hazel
1 teaspoon carrier oil
7 drops cypress essential oil
7 drops sandalwood essential oil

Combine all of the ingredients in a bowl and then transfer to the container of your choice. I recommend using this combination in a spritz bottle, but you can also "splash" it on your face as you would a normal aftershave. Just remember to shake well before using, as the contents will separate. Do not rinse off. Store in an airtight container for 6 months. Makes about 12 uses.

Bad Breath–Killing Mouthwash

The synthetic ingredients found in most conventional mouthwashes are quite harsh—bad news given that the inside of your mouth is really sensitive. In this much gentler version, antibacterial cinnamon, rosemary, and clove essential oils—which have been shown to promote dental health—provide that quintessential "fresh" feeling. Coconut oil's high levels of antimicrobial and antibacterial lauric acid make it a natural choice for this recipe.

1 tablespoon coconut oil
1 tablespoon warm water
2 drops cinnamon essential oil
2 drops rosemary essential oil
1 drop clove oil

Combine all of the ingredients in a small bowl, stirring to help the coconut oil fully liquefy. Swish about a teaspoon of liquid in your mouth as you would any other mouthwash. (It will feel weird at first, but you'll get the hang of it.) Spit out when finished. Store remaining mouthwash in an airtight container for up to 1 month. This recipe makes at least 6 uses.

SWISH AWAY

To really up your dental-hygiene game, swish the mouthwash for up to 20 minutes—it's called "oil pulling," and it's all the rage. Oil pulling helps to draw out toxins and bacteria, and may even aid in whitening teeth.

Peppermint-Clay Toothpaste

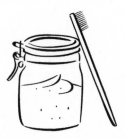

Years ago, if you told me that I'd be rubbing clay—aka *dirt*—onto my teeth to clean them, I would have laughed in your face with my fluoride-shiny teeth. But, surprise, here I am giving you the recipe for clay toothpaste that will change your world. I think bentonite clay is going to be the next big thing; it's a superhero ingredient that detoxifies, cleanses, and nourishes. Coconut oil and peppermint essential oil are both antibacterial and tremendous for dental hygiene (and coconut oil can even help whiten teeth). It may take some getting used to at first, but trust me, you'll never go back to traditional, gooey tubes of toothpaste again.

1 tablespoon coconut oil
3 tablespoons distilled water
1 tablespoon bentonite clay
4–8 drops peppermint essential oil
2–4 drops tea tree oil

Combine all of the ingredients in a bowl. Use as you would a normal toothpaste. Store in an airtight container for up to 1 week (you may need to add more water as it starts to harden). Makes about 14 uses.

BLENDS FROM THE EXPERTS

SARAH VILLAFRANCO

Sarah Villafranco is the founder and genius behind all of the beautiful formulations for Osmia Organics, a line of all-natural skincare and soaps. She also happens to be an emergency room doctor turned holistic skincare creator, so she knows what she's doing when it comes to the healing side of EOs. Sarah says, "The greatest harm you can inflict on people is allowing them to forget their own, innate power to heal their bodies and minds through the choices they make every day. When I left the practice of conventional medicine and started Osmia Organics I felt I was practicing real medicine—the kind where I can educate people, decrease the number of chemicals they use, and inspire them to heal themselves."

Here are two medicinal recipes from Sarah that you can treat as "doctor's orders."

Cold Sore Remedy

When you feel a cold sore coming on, apply a little bit of this mixture using a clean Q-Tip in the morning, and repeat as needed throughout the day. The lavender and peppermint will provide some pain relief, while the ravensara and bergamot both possess potent antiviral activity. This should reduce the duration and severity of symptoms.

1 teaspoon tamanu oil
24 drops ravensara essential oil

36 drops bergamot essential oil
12 drops lavender essential oil
12 drops peppermint essential oil

Combine all of the ingredients in a small glass bottle and shake well. Let the bottle sit in warm water for 10 minutes to allow the oils to blend thoroughly. This treatment should keep for up to 1 year. Makes about 20 uses.

Upper Respiratory Blend

This deliciously herby-smelling blend is excellent for warding off and/or alleviating cold symptoms. Basil works to reduce nervous tension and relieve headaches, while thyme and oregano are potent antibacterial weapons. Peppermint and eucalyptus loosen mucus secretions and open the airways for easier breathing, and lavender helps ease the mind and softens the medicinal scent of the blend. It is to be used via inhalation only, *not* directly on the skin.

36 drops basil essential oil
36 drops thyme essential oil
24 drops peppermint essential oil
24 drops eucalyptus essential oil
24 drops oregano essential oil
12 drops lavender essential oil

Combine all of the ingredients in a small glass bottle and shake well to combine. For best effect, use this blend in a steam shower by dropping 5–10 drops on the floor, away from any running water, where the oils can vaporize and be drawn into the respiratory system. For use on the go, put 3 drops of oil onto a tissue, and inhale deeply 5–10 times. It may also be used in a diffuser. Use this blend for up to 1 year; makes about 15 to 30 uses.

Deodorizing Underarm and Body Spray

I love a DIY cream deodorant, but I understand that some people don't enjoy applying deodorant to their underarms using their fingers. This user-friendly spray alleviates that discomfort, leveraging three deodorizing powerhouses—lavender, geranium, and patchouli—to create one potent spray (that smells amazing). Moreover, the inclusion of antibacterial olive oil means this spray won't irritate your sensitive underarms.

¼ cup distilled water
1 teaspoon olive oil
BASE NOTE: *10 drops patchouli essential oil*
MIDDLE NOTE: *10 drops geranium essential oil*
TOP NOTE: *10 drops lavender essential oil*

Combine the distilled water and olive oil in a 2-ounce glass spritz bottle. Next, add the essential oils. Shake vigorously and let sit for 48 hours before using. Spritz onto underarms, feet, or anywhere else that's kinda stinky. Store in a cool, dark place for up to 6 months. Makes at least 60 uses.

Cooling After-Sun Soak

I find that getting sunburned is not only physically painful, it's emotionally distressing, too. (I feel so irresponsible. I should know better!) Well, this soothing soak will serve as a salve for your burn *and* for your nerves. Lavender essential oil is renowned for its ability to heal burns (perhaps you recall the earlier story about chemist René-Maurice Gattefossé?) plus it will help alleviate anxiety and relax your muscles. Nourishing coconut milk will cool and hydrate your skin and witch hazel reduces inflammation. Please note that the key for this soak is to immerse yourself in *cool* water—you might shiver, but you'll feel relief!

1 can full-fat organic coconut milk
2 tablespoons witch hazel
12 drops lavender essential oil

Combine all of the ingredients in a large bowl. Fill up your bathtub with cool water. Dump half of the mixture directly into the tub and immerse yourself. Reserve the other half to pour directly onto your skin (specifically the burned areas). This recipe makes 1 use.

Mediterranean Cuticle Soak

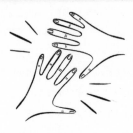

In a scene in *Mean Girls*—the 2004 Lindsay Lohan classic—actress Amanda Seyfried's character, Karen, moans, "My nail beds suck." It's a line meant to underscore the totally ridiculous ways that women pick their physical appearance apart, and while I've never given *that* much attention to my nail beds, I get that some of us struggle. This soak is great for you cuticle sufferers out there, plus it will help strengthen your nails. Lemon and myrrh essential oils are both deeply nourishing and any vitamin E–packed carrier oil will soften your skin.

2 tablespoons carrier oil
8 drops lemon essential oil
8 drops myrrh essential oil

Combine all of the ingredients in a bowl. Put one set of fingertips into the bowl and just hang out for up to 10 minutes. Repeat for the other hand. Wipe excess oil off hands. Toss after 1 use.

HOME CARE

It's easy to assume that DIY home care won't live up to the industrial-grade commercial options you're accustomed to using. But do not be fooled. Not only is the stuff at the store filled with chemicals you don't need or want in your life, I promise you it doesn't work any better than, or even as well as, these recipes. I've taken a store-bought spray and used a quarter of the bottle to clean a floor stain, while a small amount of the Grease Cleaner on page 169 works immediately, smells amazing, and doesn't make my face feel like it's burning. I fly through dish detergent in my house, but when I make the Lavender Eucalyptus Dish Soap, it lasts and lasts (and my dishes squeak). It may sound too good to be true, so you'll have to make them to see for yourself.

Not Your Average Gel Air Freshener

I cannot stand conventional air fresheners: They smell like either plastic flowers or the cheesy vanilla eau de toilette favored by seventh graders in 2002. I do, however, love the idea of gel fresheners—that "set it and forget it" mentality really appeals to my lazy side. This recipe is created using gelatin to mimic the plug-in gel packs you'd find in the home cleaning aisle. They won't fill a full room with scent, but are great for closets, bathrooms, and cars. You have some options for fragrance here, so smell as you go to see what you like!

2 cups water
¼ cup unflavored gelatin
2 tablespoons fine-grain sea salt

BASE NOTE: *20 drops frankincense essential oil*
BASE NOTE: *20 drops Peru balsam essential oil*
MIDDLE NOTE: *10 drops neroli essential oil or juniper essential oil or petitgrain essential oil*
TOP NOTE: *20 drops grapefruit essential oil or palmarosa essential oil*

In three separate small glass jars, layer the essential oil blend according to base, middle, and top notes. (Note: The quantities above represent the total needed for three gel packs, so for each container, the split should roughly be 6–7 drops frankincense, 6–7 drops Peru balsam, 3–4 drops neroli or juniper or petitgrain, and 6–7 drops grapefruit or palmarosa *in that order*.) Boil the water and add the powdered gelatin, whisking until smooth. Next, whisk in the salt, stirring until dissolved. Pour the hot gelatin on top of each combination and allow it to cool. Place wherever you want some freshening up! Makes 3 gel "packs" that will last about 2 months. If not using one, make sure to tightly seal the jar until you want to use it!

All-Purpose Counter Cleaner

This is a classic, do-it-all home cleaner. It's antibacterial, anti-microbial, antifungal, and antiseptic, and it smells great. It can be used safely on any surface, and works well on glass.

1 cup distilled water
1 teaspoon liquid castile soap (like Dr. Bronner's)
10 drops rosemary essential oil
10 drops tea tree essential oil

Combine all of the ingredients in a large spritz bottle. Shake well. Use as you would a normal cleaning spray. Will last up to 1 year and make at least 60 uses.

Lavender Eucalyptus Dish Soap

Lavender is a *great* ingredient for soap because it packs an antiseptic, antibacterial punch without being too harsh on the skin. (You won't need to wear dishwashing gloves with this one . . . not that anyone ever does anymore.) Eucalyptus is antibacterial and antifungal, but has a pretty strong, almost medicinal aroma, which is why I added sweet, floral palmarosa essential oil. It helps cut the odor a bit.

1 cup unscented liquid castile soap (like Dr. Bronner's)
1 tablespoon distilled water
15–30 drops lavender essential oil

Bad Breath–Killing
    Mouthwash, 158
Choco-Mint Dry Shampoo,
    152–53
Cold Sore Remedy, 160–61
Deodorizing Underarm and
    Body Spray, 162
Mediterranean Cuticle Soak,
    164
Nighttime Dandruff Treatment,
    154
Non-Greasy Beard Oil, 156
Peppermint-Clay Toothpaste,
    159
Rose Chamomile Conditioning
    Rinse, 155
Rosemary Clarifying Shampoo,
    151–52
Upper Respiratory Blend,
    161–62
Woodsy Witch Hazel
    Aftershave, 157
Peru balsam, 142, 166
pest spray: Catnip and Citronella
    Pest Spray, recipe, 173
petitgrain oil, 71, 166
Pharaoh Perfume, recipe, 146
phenols, 39, 42
phenylethyl alcohol, 40
phenylpropanoids, 41
photosensitive skin, 109
pine, 142
pink peppercorn oil, 147
plants:
    extracts, 12
    families of, 47–48
    spiritual connections with, 54
Pliny the Elder, Natural History, 17
pollinators, 10
potpourri, 58–59

Stovetop Essential Oil
    Potpourri, recipe, 59
pregnancy, 70–72, 92, 98
preventive care, 7, 190
primary metabolites, 9

Quick Lemongrass Bath Oil,
    recipe, 95
Quick Peppermint Lip Balm,
    recipe, 112
Quick Tea Tree Mouthwash,
    recipe, 103

ravensara oil, 160
recipes:
    All-Purpose Counter Cleaner,
        167
    Aromatic Dryer Sheets, 171–72
    Bad Breath–Killing
        Mouthwash, 158
    Beginner All-Over Lotion, 68
    Breakout Clearing Cleanser,
        129
    Candles for Four Seasons,
        174–79
    Catnip and Citronella Pest
        Spray, 173
    Choco-Mint Dry Shampoo,
        152–53
    Cold Sore Remedy, 160–61
    Cooling After-Sun Soak, 163
    Cramp Relief Oil, 97
    Deodorizing Underarm and
        Body Spray, 162
    Depression-Fighting Oil Blend,
        110
    Eucalyptus Moth Repellent, 106
    Find Your Balance Blend, 150
    Florida Face Scrub, 135
    Grease Cleaner, 169–70

recipes *(cont.)*
   Grounding Blend, 149–50
   Headache Blend, 185
   Head Cold Blend, 182–83
   Healing Blend, 149
   Indoor Forest Diffuser Blend, 108
   Lavender Eucalyptus Dish Soap, 167–68
   Lemon Pine Furniture Polish, 168–69
   Marvin Gaye Massage Oil, 139
   Mediterranean Cuticle Soak, 164
   Migraine Healing Oil, 93
   Moisturizing Spot Treatment, 138
   Motion Sickness/I-Gotta-Barf Blend, 184
   Nighttime Blend, 181
   Nighttime Dandruff Treatment, 154
   Non-Greasy Beard Oil, 156
   Not Your Average Gel Air Freshener, 165–66
   Peppermint-Clay Toothpaste, 159
   Quick Lemongrass Bath Oil, 95
   Quick Peppermint Lip Balm, 112
   Quick Tea Tree Mouthwash, 103
   Rose Chamomile Conditioning Rinse, 155
   Rosemary Clarifying Shampoo, 151–52
   Sore Throat Blend, 183
   Stop Stressing Blend, 182
   Stovetop Essential Oil Potpourri, 59
   Super Luxe Floral Face Toner, 136
   Super Simple Face Mist, 101
   Sweet-and-Spicy Body Scrub, 137
   Teatime Oily Skin Mask, 134
   Ultimate Oil Cleanser, 132
   Wake-Up Blend, 180–81
   Warm 'n' Cozy Mask, 133
   Woodsy Witch Hazel Aftershave, 157
research, 27–30
   on components, 44
   in drug testing, 28
   variables controlled in, 28
   in vitro testing, 27
Robitussin, 40
Roman chamomile oil, 71, 156
Romans, ancient, 19
rose absolute, 40, 146, 147, 150
Rose Chamomile Conditioning Rinse, recipe, 155
rose geranium, 40, 150
rosehip seed oil, 124, 132, 156
rosemary, 40, 47, 142
Rosemary Clarifying Shampoo, recipe, 151–52
rosemary oil, 20, 55–56, 73, 107–8, 152, 158, 167, 182–83
rose oil, 19, 40
rose otto, 142
rose otto oil, 71, 136, 143, 155, 176, 181
rose petals, 130
rosewater, 136

safety, 68–73
sage, 47, 70
sage oil, 67, 73, 98
sandalwood, 14, 15, 114, 142
   Sexy Sandalwood Perfume, recipe, 143

sandalwood oil, 11, 40, 71, 157
sassafras, 48
sassafras oil, 70
savory, winter, 44
savory oil, 67
scent, 12
    scent rainbow, 142
    see also perfumes
Scotch pine oil, 169
sebum, 122
secondary metabolites, 10
sesame oil, 67, 125
sesquiterpene alcohols, 40, 42
sesquiterpenes, 39, 42
Sexy Sandalwood Perfume, recipe, 143
shea butter, 68
Sina, Ali ibn, 18
skin:
    allergic reactions of, 65, 69
    dermal sensitization, 69–70, 92
    direct application to, 66
    photosensitive, 109
    and prescription medications, 70
    sensitive, 66
    specific benefits to, 67
    testing for, 120, 127
skincare products, 66–67, 128–39
    Breakout Clearing Cleanser, 129
    Florida Face Scrub, 135
    Marvin Gaye Massage Oil, 139
    Moisturizing Spot Treatment, 138
    Super Luxe Floral Face Toner, 136
    Sweet-and-Spicy Body Scrub, 137
    Teatime Oily Skin Mask, 134
    Ultimate Oil Cleanser, 132

Warm 'n' Cozy Mask, 133
skin cleanse: Ultimate Oil Cleanser, recipe, 132
Skin Cleanse (Grigore), xi
solvent extraction, 78–79, 123
Sore Throat Blend, recipe, 183
spas, 24
spearmint, 40, 47, 50
spearmint oil, 184
spicy scents, 142
Spring: Floral Hothouse candle, 174, *175*, 176
spruce oil, 39
star anise oil, 67
starch, 9
steam distillation, 9, 19, 75–76, 77
Stop Stressing Blend, recipe, 182
Stovetop Essential Oil Potpourri, recipe, 59
stress: Stop Stressing Blend recipe, 182
stress hormones, 56
Summer: Vanilla Citronella candle, 174, *175*, 177
sunburn, 163
supercritical (CO2) extraction, 79
Super Luxe Floral Face Toner, recipe, 136
Super Simple Face Mist, recipe, 101
S.W. Basics, xii, xvii, 24
sweet almond oil, 121
Sweet-and-Spicy Body Scrub, recipe, 137
sweet basil oil, 67
sweet birch oil, 67
sweet marjoram oil, 71
sweet orange oil, 109–10, 145, 149–50
    Depression-Fighting Oil Blend recipe, 110

tagetes oil, 67
tamanu oil, 160
tangerine, 47
tangerine oil, 133
Teatime Oily Skin Mask, recipe, 134
tea tree, 48, 142
tea tree oil, 102–4
    components of, 45, 46
    health benefits of, 67, 102–3, 154
    in recipes, 103, 129, 154, 159, 167
    safety of, 71
thyme, 47, 142
thyme oil, 39, 67, 70, 156, 161
thymol, 44
Tisserand, Robert, 191
trade secrets, 32
transpiration, 11
tuberose, 80
turmeric, 15, 40, 48
turmeric oil, 39

Ultimate Oil Cleanser, recipe, 132
unrefined oils, 121
Upper Respiratory Blend, recipe, 161–62
USDA Organic Program, 82, 120

Valnet, Jean, 22
Vanilla Citronella candle, 174, *175*, 177

vanillin, 40
variability, 29
vetiver, 142, 145
Vicks VapoRub, 6
Villafranco, Sarah, 160
vitamin K, 47
volatile components, 12

Wake-Up Blend, recipe, 180–81
Warm 'n' Cozy Mask, recipe, 133
Wasfie, Giselle, 16
water, distilled, 140
white lotus absolute, 146
white pine, 19
"wildcrafted," 82
wild things, 83
Winter: Classic Holiday candle, 174, *175*, 179
wintergreen oil, 67
witch hazel, 11, 163, 173
woodsy scents, 142
Woodsy Witch Hazel Aftershave, recipe, 157
word of mouth advertising, 33
World War II, treating injuries in, 22
wormwood oil, 70

ylang ylang, 41, 56, 71, 139, 142, 171
Young Living, 23
yuzu oil, 181

About the Author

ADINA GRIGORE is the author of *Skin Cleanse* and the founder and CEO of the all-natural, sustainable skincare line S.W. Basics, which she started out of her kitchen in 2011. A graduate of the Institute for Integrative Nutrition, Adina has worked in the wellness industry since 2007 as a private holistic nutrition-ist, a personal trainer, and a workshop coordinator teaching people about the DIY nature of wellness. S.W. Basics products are now sold internationally and have been featured in *Vogue*, *O, The Oprah Magazine*, *W Magazine*, the *New York Times*, *In-Style*, *Real Simple*, and *Martha Stewart Living*, among other pub-lications.

ALSO BY ADINA GRIGORE

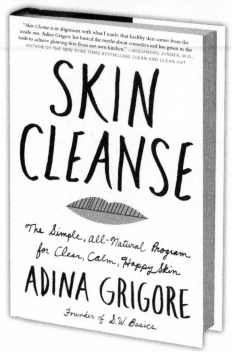

SKIN CLEANSE
The Simple, All-Natural Program for Clear, Calm, Happy Skin
Available in Hardcover and E-book

"*Skin Cleanse* is in alignment with what I teach: that healthy skin comes from the inside out. Adina Grigore has busted the myths about cosmetics and has given us the tools to achieve glowing skin from our own kitchen."
—Alejandro Junger, M.D., *New York Times* bestselling author of *Clean and Clean Gut*

The secret to beautiful skin is simple: it's an inside job.

In *Skin Cleanse*, Adina Grigore explains how the state of your skin is a direct reflection of what's going on inside of your body. *Skin Cleanse* helps readers diagnose and understand the underlying causes of their individual skin problems and offers all-natural recipes—using inexpensive ingredients that can be found at the grocery store—to treat them effectively. With a step-by-step skin detox as well targeted solutions for specific skin concerns such as dryness, oiliness, and acne, Grigore empowers you with the information you need to take control over your skin once and for all.

Available Wherever Books Are Sold

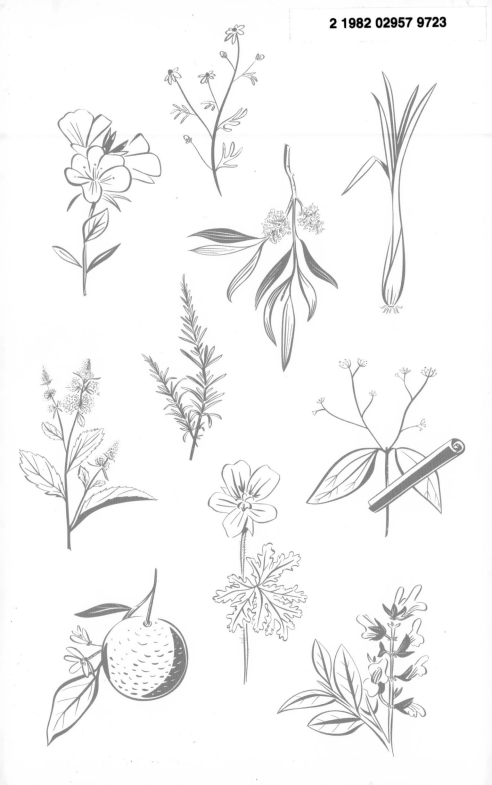